AHIMSA

BUDDHISM
AND THE VEGETARIAN IDEAL

Revised Edition

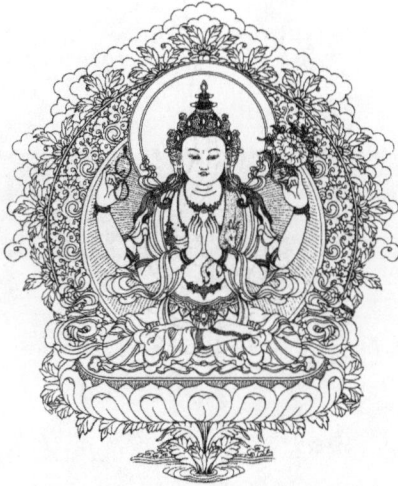

BODO BALSYS

UNIVERSAL DHARMA
PUBLICATIONS
SYDNEY, AUSTRALIA

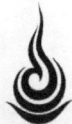

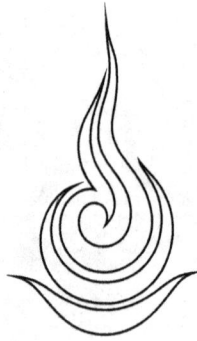

ISBN   978-0-6487877-5-4

© 2024 Balsys, Bodo
Revised Edition of 2004 publication
Updated 2026

Dedication

Obeisance to the Gurus.

Oṁ

Thanks to Laura Inwood, Ruth Fitzpatrick, Angie O'Sullivan, Rob MacDonald and Kylie Smith for their assistance.

Contents

Preface

❀

The overarching purpose of this book is to better inform those Buddhists that consume their brothers of the animal kingdom as to why they should refrain.

I apologise for any inner turmoil that may be evoked within the reader in response to the content of this short treatise. However, by reading this book, such readers are at least considerate enough to care. In any case, if emotions are stirred and the immediate (albeit transient) pain is enough to produce a change in awareness within the reader that saves the life of even one animal, then this writing will not be in vain.

I understand that there are many social mores and customs indoctrinated into people of all backgrounds. These are generally well entrenched and accordingly govern the lives of those born into that society. This does not mean that change is not possible, and indeed history abounds with the stories of meaningful changes that have perpetually arisen within all societies. Change is inevitable, being one of the key pillars of the *buddhadharma*. Indeed, change must occur in an arena of immediate, compassionate concern related to meat consumption. There are many reasons for this, as will be shown.

This writing is dedicated to all those who are willing to think and act compassionately. Its focus is necessarily slanted towards Tibetan Buddhist monks because they have set their sights high in spreading their *dharma* to the West. Thus inadvertently (and rightfully) have purported themselves as teachers in many arenas. Their rich culture and teachings on wisdom and compassion are examples that many in the West are inspired by, apart from the major problem of a seemingly hypocritical stance regarding their animal brothers.

If Tibetans wish to rightly educate people about ethics, then all forms of hypocrisy must go. They must therefore sacrifice aspects of their customs and personal desires in relation to their eating habits. They would then be setting an admirable example, sounding out a great message for the world at large. This is particularly important for the ever-growing number of Western Buddhists who continue to seek guidance from their Tibetan teachers and who inevitably pose the question: 'Should we be vegetarian?' This would heal a great wound being carved by the erroneous responses presently being given to them.

If we are to root out all ignorance, we must rightly educate all who seek to develop *bodhicitta*.[1] Rather than encouraging apathy through submissive responses, let us deliver the message loudly and clearly that needless killing and suffering is wrong. In doing so, let us begin to awaken the gateways of compassionate understanding in the whole of humanity. Let us work to create a world where needless killing does not occur. This work must start with the most loving and compassionate beings on earth – those whom have devoted their existence to relieve the suffering of all sentient beings. They are those that have placed the evocation of harmlessness and compassion at the forefront of their lives. As we strive to relieve all forms of suffering (that being the greatest calling of our lives), let us provide to each other all the necessary encouragement, knowledge and insight to do so.

This book is in the form of a compassionate plea that calls upon Buddhists to utilise their power and influence to the greatest means possible. So may it be that our compassionate understanding is expanded and the strength and power of the Buddha's way is purified and energised for millennia to come.

May we all continue to grow infinitely in wisdom and compassion and walk the Bodhisattva Way.

Oṁ Maṇi Vajrapāni Hūṁ!

---

1   *Bodhicitta* can be translated as the consciousness of compassion. It can be conceived of as the compassionate force that propels one towards gaining enlightenment.

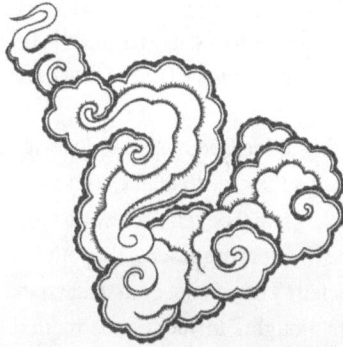

1

The Harmfulness of Meat-Eating

The eating of meat cannot in any way be considered to be helpful to the practice of the *dharma*. Neither can the slaughter of animals be considered to be consistent with the Buddhist teachings of loving-kindness, harmlessness, compassion *(mettā, ahiṃsā, karuṇā),* or the development of the enlightenment-Mind via the evocation of *bodhicitta.* The cruelties associated with the slaughter of the animal kingdom for human consumption (pain, fear, and the distress suffered in the process of being fattened for butchering), as well as the environmental disasters wreaked upon our planet through the meat industry, are well documented. Such concepts should be properly considered by all claiming to be developing *bodhicitta.* Although there are now many books on the subject, we also have statements purported to have been said by the Buddha, such as in *The Śūraṅgama Sūtra,* which states:

The reason for practicing dhyāna and seeking to attain Samādhi is to escape from the suffering of life, but in seeking to escape from suffering ourselves why should we inflict it upon others? Unless you can so control your minds that even the thought of brutal unkindness and killing is abhorrent, you will never be able to escape from the bondage of the world's life...After my Parinirvāṇa in the last kalpa different kinds of ghosts will be encountered everywhere deceiving people and teaching them that they can eat meat and still attain enlightenment...How can a bhikṣhu, who hopes to become a deliverer of others, himself be living on the flesh of other sentient beings?[1]

It is thus astounding to see Buddhists eating meat, and *yet in the name of teaching compassion* they try to alter their values in the spirit of the Western revolution of critical thought. So why do those who are spiritually orientated follow the illogical arguments that our Western brothers who eat meat have concocted? They do not even understand the environmental effects of how their thoughts influence the mental atmosphere of all beings in the world at large; environmental effects are conditioned by thought, and these thoughts are cloudy and uncompassionate.

When formerly living in Tibet, the climatic conditions were severe, making the eating of grazing animals a viable necessity for some Buddhists. The animals were slaughtered with respect, and veneration for the sacredness of Life was upheld. Now Tibetans have monasteries in India where they live with our vegetarian Hindu spiritual brothers, and clearly have no need to eat meat.

Thus their continued eating of grazing animals is no longer viable, nor is it necessary. Often the Buddhist mind is too grey to perceive the illogicality of continued meat consumption, and the urgent need to alter this custom's trend. Their attitudes towards eating meat are staunchly entrenched. They work hard to preserve the habits of older thinking, despite the added pressure of publicly giving teachings to the West. The immorality is even more apparent due to examples of the modern modes of mass slaughter of animals for the consumption of meat (displaying to us so clearly the cruelty of this habit). It is not just a relatively few animals taken from the wild anymore, as the Tibetans

---

1   Version from: *A Buddhist Bible,* ed. Dwight Goddard (New York: Dutton. 1952), 264-5.

once did, it is billions of sentient lives slaughtered yearly. Compassion dictates these species should be protected – preserved, intact and alive.

One can ask, how can you truly be a spiritual being when you help kill animals through the eating of meat? Your intention to not harm is negated by your intention to eat meat. Therefore, you are the perpetrator of suffering upon others. Your Buddhist vows are useless, 'let suffering rule the world' you inadvertently say as you eat the cow. You are effectively killing in the name of your spirituality, as if your *dharma* is clean. Spirituality starts to be defiled not only when the knife comes down upon the lamb but by one's intention to provide patronage to the butcher shop, wherein the killing has been done for you.

Buddhists who wish to justify meat eating often state that the Buddha said in the *Jīvaka Sutta:* 'that in three cases meat must not be eaten: if it has been seen, heard, or suspected that it was intended for the person'.[2] It should however be noted that this statement was given by the Buddha solely because of the problem faced by ordained monks when begging for food, and being given meals containing meat by their hosts. Rather than reject what was given to them (a charitable intention, generative of good *karma* for that individual), the Buddha said that they would eat only under the strict conditions mentioned above, 'without being fettered and infatuated'. By the last statement, the Buddha regarded the mind's non-attachment to whatever came to a monk as most important, thus to being non-attached to what food one ate, or being infatuated with food.

Of course, the Buddhist may say that he can eat meat without being fettered to the thought of so eating (etc.), but could s/he also do so if

---

2   The entire conversation reads thus: "Jivaka told Buddha that he had heard that people killed living things intending them for Buddha, and that he ate the meat prepared on that account. He asked if such persons were truth-speakers and did not accuse the Lord falsely. Buddha replied that it was not true, but that in three cases meat must not be eaten: if it has been seen, heard, or suspected that it was intended for the person. If a monk who practises the brahma-vihara of love accepts an invitation in a village, he does not think, "verily this house-holder is providing me with excellent food; may he provide me with excellent food in the future." "He eats the food without being fettered in the future." "He eats the food without being fettered and infatuated." "What do you think, Jivaka, does the monk at that time think of injury to himself, to others, or to both?" "Certainly not, Lord." "Does not a monk at that time take blameless food?" *Jivaka Sutta* (M.N.I. 368). Quoted from: *A Comparative Study of Jainism and Buddhism*, by Brahmcahri Sital Prashad, 246-7.

what was offered to be eaten was direct poison? Does not what one consumes directly affect the physical body and mind, despite one's ability to rightly meditate? One must give a thought as to the type of life one is to live and for the road to enlightenment ahead. One must think clearly on what is consumed, or any other type of action that one might do, as to the harm it may or may not cause the body, mind, or to other sentient beings. If one does not do so, and yet claims to be 'unfettered', then this claim is foolish. Indeed, one may become very much fettered to the continuous *karma*-producing actions that myopic self-deceptive thoughts will surely produce. It is like putting a blanket over one's head and then claiming that the darkness that one sees is *nirvāṇa*.

The only proper way to interpret the Buddha's statement above (from a Mahāyāna perspective) is that the consumption of meat was not at all agreeable to the Buddha or to his disciples, and he would rather them abstain altogether. However, the practice of begging for alms (in an unfettered manner) required a consideration of the merit of the kind donor offering food. By accepting food from the donor, the monk would facilitate the production of a good karmic/dharmic connection with that person. This could grow in future lives to be a positive interaction, as the monk evolves upon the Bodhisattva path (to eventually become a Buddha).

The offering of food by laypeople also allowed a possible discourse from the monks on the *buddhadharma*. The possibility of this type of good *karma* being denied (if the *bhikṣu* rejected the food offering from the host) had to be weighed up against the ideal of strict vegetarianism. Nevertheless, the spirit of the Buddha's teaching is clear – do not eat meat if it is in any way avoidable. If monks accepted meat products in foods under the guidelines set out by the Buddha (i.e., 'if it has been seen, heard, or suspected that it was intended for the person'), their *karma* with the animal kingdom would be counterbalanced with the good *karma* gained by the interrelation with the host. In our consideration, the term 'unfettered' really means that which leads to the walking of the Bodhisattva path and consequent Buddhahood.

In any case, the *Jīvaka Sutta* is Theravādin, and later Mahāyāna texts, such as the *Śūraṅgama* and *Laṅkāvatāra Sūtras* made it very clear that eating meat was wrong and totally unacceptable.

Monks used to literally roam the country begging for alms, and this was the way they ate, thus the rule was to accept what you were given. However, the truth of the matter is that now it is rare to find Buddhist monks of the Mahāyāna schools begging for alms or food. They are given money or alms and are fed thereby. Thus they have the option now to truly exercise their compassion (by being selective as to what they buy to eat), yet many continue to buy meat. To properly follow the teachings of the Buddha, one must neither purchase meat nor consume it. One's intention must not be the consuming of meat that has been slaughtered for oneself (or for the monastery).

By analysing the Buddha's statement, 'if it has been seen, heard, or suspected that it was intended for the person', in the modern day context, we see that many monks in fact violate all three rules.

1. It matters little whether the butcher knows or does not know who is purchasing the meat, he knows that the monks in the monastery eat meat and that is a good enough cause to kill the animal. He will kill because he has seen 'you', that is 'a' or any number of Buddhist monks patronising his shop. It does not matter which of 'you' comes to buy the meat for the monastery.

2. In the present day case, the monks go directly to a butcher to purchase with full knowledge of the fact that they are to buy a carcass that they will consume, thereby producing direct *karma* with the animals. The butcher has heard the monks asking for meat, therefore he supplies it to them. They have heard that his prices are the cheapest, therefore they will patronise. The butcher has heard the monk's request for cheaper meat and to compete with other butchers makes the produce of slaughter more competitive. Thus the story runs in our societies. Whether the purchaser be monks or laity purchasing for monks matters little in this equation.

3. The servant of the Monastery sent to purchase the food thus goes directly to the killer, whom from then on suspects with some certainty that he will return to purchase the products of the butchery.

We see in the above that many present day monks do not at all follow the spirit of the Buddha's concession to his monks, or the nature of *ahiṃsā*. Such actions cannot, therefore, be properly justified by any twist of the imagination.

What we are essentially talking about is a very basic law, that of supply and demand. If there is no need (demand) for umbrellas because it ceases to rain, then the supply will quickly cease also. Similarly, if no meat eaters exist (i.e., if the human race became vegetarian) then there would be no need to kill animals for food. The demand would cease and thus the supply would also cease to be. People would then get all of their nutritional supplies from pulses, vegetables, nuts, and fruits. Greater demand would produce an improved supply of vegetarian staples, replacing the uneconomical and environmentally destructive process of supplying carcasses to eat. No one would be motivated to supply dead animals. As such, generations of these creatures would be relieved of undeserved suffering. The shepherd would become a soybean farmer and so on, producing the ramifications of expansive good will and compassion throughout society. The butcher would cease to exist.

One can also look at this from a slightly different viewpoint. There is a law in the West that makes the receiving of stolen goods illegal. By making this illegal, it essentially stops or limits the thief's ability to capitalise on his/her crimes. There is no similar law that prohibits the butcher from selling his/her goods, thus animals needlessly die due to the views and commonplace attitudes of people whom willingly purchase flesh. They see only a product, not the life of the animal and why it was killed. There is another parallel between meat consumerism and the process of thieving. If you have possessions in a house and you get burgled, then part of the pain is the cost of having to replace what was taken. The animal (once consumed) must be replaced, and this is the pain of the animal kingdom – the continual replacement of slaughtered animals by new animals for human consumption. People don't just kill once, they kill again and again. Thieves don't just steal once if they can get away with it, they steal again and again. The receiver of stolen goods rewards the thief for thievery, as does the meat eater reward the butcher for killing. Just because you didn't kill the animal yourself doesn't make it right to subscribe to the killing of animals.

So, how many more generations of animals (i.e., how many billions of future individual animal units) need to get slaughtered because of this 'replacement factor'? This is a contemplation that many Buddhists have not yet thought about.

You have been killing and maiming animals for years and have not seen that commerce, as we call it in the West, means cause and effect, supply and demand. Some people steal possessions only because demand is there, which incentivises them to achieve access. Making a parallel between the *karma* of killing and the *karma* of stealing means that both animals and property are only interfered with if another group of people are willing to pay for that product. The understanding as to how *karma* works here is simple.

The laws of our societies are made to prevent stealing from within,[3] as much as possible. To prevent animals from being killed, consumers must radically change their dietary preferences, and consider the argument of pain and suffering to avoid further harm.

Many Buddhists also look to the way the Buddha is purported to have died as another excuse for eating meat. It should be noted that the Buddha didn't necessarily eat pig meat when he died; it can also be argued that he ate "a poisonous truffle (a species of mushroom)".[4]

---

3   If caught, the thief often denies that he stole, in a similar way that meat eaters often deny that they cause any harm. Stealing from within, refers in part to, internally lying to oneself that meat eating/stealing is justifiable, despite what they know in conscience to be true.

4   This is explained in detail on pp. 23-35 in the book *To Cherish all Life* by Roshi Philip Kapleau. Part of what he states is:

In view of the first precept's prohibition against causing another to take life, it is appropriate to inquire how meat-eating Buddhist priests, monks, and teachers justify such a transgression. Question them and they are sure to say, "Don't you know that the Buddha himself ate a piece of pork offered to him at the home of one of his followers? Although normally he did not eat flesh foods, his sense of gratitude would not permit him to refuse it. Like the Buddha, we gratefully eat whatever is put before us, without preference or aversion"...And then they will add, "And are you not also aware that the Buddha laid down the rule that one must refrain from meat eating only if one knows, hears, or suspects the animal has been killed specifically for one's own consumption?".....monks, teachers and lay people have taken refuge in these supposed actions and statements of the Buddha to justify their meat eating, implying that if the Buddha himself ate flesh foods when it was offered to him, surely they have warrant to do likewise. What they gloss over with respect to the first proposition is the research of scholars, the majority of whom contend that it was not a piece of

But the symbolism of eating meat, here as 'pig meat', being deadly to the human form is correct. Why was the symbolism (rightly utilised by thinking Buddhists as a reason not to eat meat) used to justify their morally bankrupted actions (i.e., consuming their defenceless cousins)?

Could you chomp on a living animal? If not, your desire to eat meat means you have to kill first, so that it doesn't wriggle about, and you don't have to be peeved by the truth. Meat eaters would discover the truth of animal suffering if they actually had to slaughter each animal first before consumption. In future lives, *karma* dictates that all the sickness you have caused by your desires to kill will descend upon you. Objectively, the suffering will be in a different form than that of the animal slaughtered, but for the senses (subjectively) the experience will be a closer approximation. You will be experiencing exactly what harm you caused in another's life by your previous desirous consumption. The karmic reality of the suffering you have caused will be yours to experience in the future. There is little difference whether it resolves in this or that life, but Buddhists should aim to transcend suffering by breaking free of those activities which cause harm to others, and thus from having to incarnate again to pay back the *karma* in a future life.

Attacks of sickness are but the *karma* of paying for former life activities, of making others suffer as a consequence of your actions. Many human sicknesses are the result of the killing of innocent animals and of their meat ingestion.

Indeed, sickness is largely the result of general emotionality, and also of killing - of other humans in former lives, of destroying of that which is good and healthy in our societies, and similarly in each individual

---

meat but a poisoned truffle (a species of mushroom) that caused the Buddha's death, and what they ignore with respect to the second are the Mahâyâna scriptures, which unequivocally condemn meat eating.

Kapleau then goes into the scholarly research and ends with:

Laying aside scholarship, what reasonable person can believe that Chunda offered the Buddha a piece of pork when the latter came to pay him a visit? As one of the Buddha's followers, surely he would have known that flesh food was not part of the Buddha's diet. (Very likely Chunda didn't eat meat himself, as most Indians still don't today.) Why, then, would he have offered meat to the World-Honoured One, a person so sensitive to the sufferings of all living beings that he would not drink milk from a cow during the first ten days after its calf was born?

human unit. It really concerns the killing or maiming of the principle of *bodhicitta*. Where *bodhicitta* is stifled and denied, there is a cause of ailment, suffering.

Your belly is the gravestone that displays the reasons for the killing. Therein lies the *karma* of the living and the dead. As a meat consumer, you are a walking mass grave. You own all the actions that produced the bones, clean and white. Each gravestone has all the records of *karma* imprinted upon it, the reasons for death, the names of the animals that died, the society in question, and the particular being who ate them.

Bulldozers of realisations gradually come to the ignorant. They retrieve the bones in order to find the cause. What was the cause of 'its' death you ask, as you hold the bone up? Its cause is a society (or any particular individual) that chooses to nourish their bodies by killing animals (beings less worthy of life in their eyes). People have no right to judge; all Life is precious. The gravestones made of the bones celebrate the burial of common sense, ignoring the logicality of a vegetarian diet.

To be a loving being one must love only the *dharma*. 'Dharma' means that meat eating Buddhist monks have to reincarnate to cleanse the *karma* of meat consumption. To do so, they must then educate others (in non hypocritical ways) as to the nature of the pain caused by such acts. This means that the breath of Life sucked from the animal is atoned for (consolidated) by the fact that those that killed will reserve similar *karma*. The light shines on. Buddhists: darn your socks, there are holes in your logic – the logic that must support your feet for the walking to enlightenment.

We expect more Buddhists to be vegetarians. Today we need more examples of vegetarianism, and Buddhists who are pledged to be so. In the world of spirituality, we receive impressions/visions via the third Eye and see that the aura of the Buddhist community is not clear or clean. They should be making an example of true spirituality for the world at large. Radiance is what we expect from those who aspire for the Bodhisattva path (not the dull auras caused by consumption of meat *prāṇās*).[5]

---

5   The vital or psychic energy in the body that vitalises all aspects of it. There are five different types of *prāṇa*, which are explained in my revised book *The Revelation*.

You enslave animals by your will to eat meat. Your carnal desire lassos their necks with every thought of supper. How can you fry one in the pan without enslaving your desires to it? You have cheated it of its life and paid for it in money; how can you expect the good *karma* of coming back a sage (for example) when you have fortified your desires around the carnal act of killing? Your good Buddhist *dharma* and ego for spiritual life is just that of enslavement of bodily form to meat, and your desires voraciously manifest as the hunter. The hunt for meat is the intent to kill. How can an animal not suffer with your desire to eat meat? The animal must suffer – if you eat meat you have killed. It is of little worth if you've got someone else to do that killing for you because of the society you live in. Essentially the *karma* is the same, it is that of intent to harm, and this is followed through by the law of *karma*. (By 'intent to harm' I mean that the truth is that your intention *is to* harm an animal, even though you may lie to yourself that this is not so, inventing all types of excuses as to why eating meat is justifiable.) The irrevocable fact is that the animal is killed because of your actions. It is harmed as its life is prematurely curtailed.

An animal someone kills you'll eat, and whatever animal you eat you've essentially killed. (This is a simple equation of the direct sequence of events surrounding the butcher's shop.) The same goes with accepting meat from families that feed you (whether through begging or by being a member of that family). Inadvertently, if with this 'acceptance' you put your 'feelings of compassion' out into society, you still cannot help the butcher who is indirectly employed by you to kill, to slaughter, since your compassion cannot help the death of that one innocent animal amongst many. Maybe you are 'compassionate', but its suffering is nonetheless yours. For this reason you are karmically indebted.

The killer has his sights on all humans in the local area where he intends to sell meat. Therefore, when meat is sold the expectation is of a human intending to eat it, be it fish,[6] sheep, cow, goat or pig. It is killed so that you are able to eat it. If he did not kill it, it would not be offered

---

6   Fish/seafood are sentient creatures with a nervous system and thus feel pain when caught, so they come under the general heading of 'meat'. However, they may have a higher energy field than grazing animals, thus being a little cleaner (energy wise) for human consumption.

by your family (or the family that hosts you). Therefore when you agree to the contract of eating meat, you agree to the killing of the animal - you are condoning the custom of meat, of killing for consumption.

This unthinking 'acceptance' of families also means that children are automatically fed meat and meat products, and are educated to think that this is a worthwhile practice. Consequently, this harm (of false beliefs) is perpetuated in our societies through many generations. As a karmic consequence, myriads of sentient beings suffer and sickness is perpetuated everywhere.

We can also look at a hypocritical culture, where the young deer or lamb is worshipped as a childhood 'darling'.[7] In effect, what happens to these animals (these 'heroes', if you like) are the procedures of the meat industry; canned, crushed and made into little fixations of 'I like this and that', in terms of meat and meat products. Does childhood love deserve such disrespect? Children do not determine what fodder they will have to eat, it is forced upon them by unthinking adults. Such enforcement of insensate eating practices must go. It tramples upon the sensitive psyche of children and corrupts their love for animals. They should instead be taught the *bodhicitta* way.

The term 'I love animals' does not personify the experience – to truly love something means to preserve it at all costs in the form it was intended. (Thus the idolised animal form, and not the can of meat, or meat product, which is presumed worthy for human consumption.)

Free the cattle, liberate the children from ungainly thoughts, teach them the truth by unveiling the images of animal suffering, and make the vegetable gardens grow. Tell the children: 'I will not have a hand in the meat industry, or an intent to kill, and when I see meat on other's tables, I will not condone their intent to kill either'.

Do we bring babies into manifestation just to kill them in later life, and expect them to thank us for a plan to bring them into incarnation? Do we give them a pre-worked out life length in unison with the joys of conscious experience until that point in time when we choose to exterminate them in the way that we currently treat animals? No race of animals (or indeed, any woman or man) at the point of pre-incarnation

---

7 As is 'Bambi', the famous Walt Disney character. Such imagery is also given to us in the Jatāka tales where the Buddha often sacrificed his life for the sake of animals.

would be happy to think 'how marvellous' it was that they would get a pre-ordained timed period to fit their life into before they are slaughtered. The decision to slaughter basically stems from people's projected ownership over cows, sheep, etc. If they applied this logic in deciding to have babies, then they should be able to kill their children at a certain date as a consequence of determining the fate of their possessions.

I am overjoyed that at least mothers do not think of their children in the way that they think of some animals. Is this because they love them? By extension, we may see that meat eating Buddhists, for all intents and purposes, do not love animals as much as they claim. Subjectively, what differentiates animals from humans in this consideration? Compassion, as a law of Love, may blend and heal their wounds of unlovingness. If there is no 'I' at the centre of being (according to Buddhist philosophy) between the species of man and that of a creature such as a dog, then what differentiates humans from animals and the way one would treat either species? The Buddhist explorers of universal Love and consciousness might learn a thing or two from human psychology (i.e., the motives for killing, and the motives for not killing, in accordance *with* the law of Love) if they reflected more upon why they consume meat. They should note that the same type of Love, as a justifiable effect, stops a mother from pre-planning a determined life span for her child or children.

Meat eating has been described to us as unfavourable in Buddhism mainly because of the suffering caused. Yet, 'how many millions of Buddhists survive on the slaughter of the beloveds?' we ask. If all those Buddhists, individually and in groups, eat and consume meat products, then in terms of *karma,* those Buddhists (who should be living examples of compassion for the world) are killing animals. For compassionate individuals, the empathetic response will be automatic when they view the bleeding ventricles of an animal falling on the floor. They could imagine that the creature's last thought as it dies is asking, 'why, what for?' Would animals think, 'well Mr. butcher/consumer/Lama, you are a saviour with a knife, but what a cruel saviour you are, that you would take any life away for your greedy purpose'.

Shame, shame on you out there! I say shame on you for not producing *karma* of a good kind. You Buddhists should know better, and those of you who actually are vegetarians should at least try to educate your fellow brothers who fall into this karmic hell-producing form of action. It's within your spiritual teachings to realise the empirical laws of *karma,* and you should meditate on them well. You have forgotten the cow and how it lives in your belly of discontent (its death and the resulting burial in your stomach) as you contentedly meditate on the reasons for life and suffering. The cow suffers in the throes of death because of your consumption, and their fear is *prāṇa* you have ingested into your constitution. It becomes part of your aggregates, the *skandhas* and *saṃskāras*[8] that you will carry on to future lives. Why can't you leave animals alone in the fields? Why do you have to employ the butcher to chop your meat? How can you thus love the cow, as you should, as well as all other animals and products of Nature? You symbolically sit in a jail with the horse of mind wondering why one suffers, with your *karma* of death and the suffering of animals resting in your belly.

Clean up your meat eating *saṃskāras* (you, the one who meditates on 'suffering'), otherwise you will suffer the *karma* of killing, and it is deadly. For you have already inadvertently chosen so to die. Get back to basics, go to a pro-vegetarian diet, to eating the vegetables that have evolved to be consumed by the animal kingdom as part of their evolutionary thrust. Get on with life so that you won't consume and create so much *karma.* If Buddhists truly loved, as they should according to the doctrine of *bodhicitta,* then much sickness would be ameliorated and premature death for the Life principle ended. For, the agonising throes of death are synonymous with those of the animals that you have caused to die prematurely. Thus you linger in cycles of pain before you die. You are always looking to the causes of suffering, so what are the chains of action that prove repetitive incarnation necessary? Myriads are held thus in thrall.

You have to look at your belly to see why you have caused so much pain to others, keeping the chains intact. You are suffering and yet you make another suffer. You, the teaching element, are actually teaching the butcher to kill for your supper, so you can eat meat. Your responsibility, however, is to rightly teach the butcher, to show wisdom, to explain that the cutting down of a lamb is aggressive. Instead, you sing praises to

---

8   Volitional tendencies developed in each life. See my book *Karma and the Rebirth of Consciousness* for a complete description of these.

the butcher that it is fine. Your selfish mentality betrays the life of the lamb and also the *lack* of knowledge of the teacher. What is expected of you is to teach the butcher 'do not kill', for it is a bloody affair. The consumption of animals means death, nothing less. Do not destroy the vital principles of life; abstain from eating animals, fellow earth dwellers. Those with little sense and with common abilities see not the harm it causes to the human and the animal body incarnated into (for both are one). Those that read these words, however, should have a far greater sophisticated aptitude for clear reasoning. Therefore, clean your plate of the filthy swine (or the mutton, etc.) and move on. You are not about meat eating, you are about Love, and for that you are truly grateful. If you eat animals that harm you not, then the lamb's leg harvested by the abattoir procedures remains your *karma*. If you cannot abstain from the flesh of others then I have reason to believe you have not fully understood *karma,* or its definition.[9] You are succumbing to the world's callous, ignorant attitudes towards the mass slaughter of animals – producing the *saṃskāras* of an appetite for meat and blood.

This only proves that Buddhists who eat meat had previous lives as non-Buddhists, where the concept of *ahiṃsā* was not part of the cultural norm and those *saṃskāras* have been brought through to this life. One should not persist in further engendering such *saṃskāras* when clearly Buddhist education gives the unique opportunity to cleanse them once and for all, and to thereby firmly set one's feet upon the Bodhisattva path. Otherwise, why pretend to be a Buddhist, where compassion for all sentient beings is taught? Fix up your *saṃskāras* and actually follow the *buddhadharma* (as it was intended by the Buddha for you to do).

---

9   People's hazy understanding of the doctrine of *karma* is where the real problem lies. This is a subject of such great import that it is discussed in detail in my book *Karma and the Rebirth of Consciousness*. There is also a brief explanation of *karma* in Appendix II.

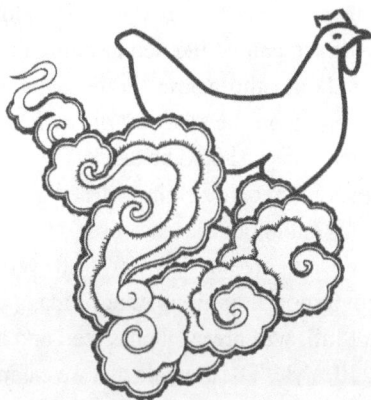

2

War upon the Animal Kingdom

We can liken the perpetual and regimental killing of animals to a war. From an animal's perspective, this would be self-evident. If the chicken had a voice, then it would reassure us that it had no self-defence or defensive mechanism against human predation. This is especially so when considering modern mass factory farming methods, where millions of chickens destined for slaughter are couped up in tiny spaces in appalling conditions. This is reminiscent of a situation far worse for chickens than the concentration camps in World War II were for humans. (At least there was an eventual end to that slaughter of human forms, but not so for chickens.) The killing only increases.

A war between animals and men, where one side is killing, and the other not so, can be likened to the invasion of Tibet by China.[1] Where is human spirituality amidst this fetish for killing? In this analogy, China stands for the idea of the killer, and the lamb (or China's fodder, that which is killed) is Tibet. There was no attempt to intervene (by the World) in China's then slaughter of a religion and its followers. Cultural genocide in a slow form can be likened to humanity's manipulation of animals. Animals are the prime target (as were Tibetans) for mistreatment – stepping on the territory of the body, squeezing the life out, where no such steps should be taken.

Certainly, to prevent people's rightful freedom of expression is a criminal activity. 'What about that of animals?'. In a society where animals, or the innocent, are cut down or destroyed without justice, then those with high moral opinions (that propagate harmlessness), or those that won't kill, will always be berated and marginalised for their peace loving lifestyle. The animals that we eat mean us no harm; they are non-aggressive, with no intent to even interact with humans.

---

1   In this text, due to the focus on Tibetan Buddhism, China's conquest of Tibet and the karmic implications are indicated. However, the purpose is not to vilify or focus prejudicially on China based on these historical events. Despite the invasion of Tibet, many positive steps forward within China over the past half century can be noted that have dramatically improved the quality of life of her citizens. Such progress includes bringing approximately 800 million people out of poverty and into relative economic prosperity. Also, public services (such as education, health care, transportation, scientific research facilities, utilities and access to the internet) have been dramatically improved. China has become a frequent target of lying Western mass media campaigns denoting it as a threat to world peace. This can be largely attributed to the unipolar American hegemony that fears the rise of China as a harbinger of the coming multi-polar era of political and interrelated economic relations. The emergence of China as a rising power, counterbalancing overt Western dominance, helps to curb American tendencies towards unilateral militaristic endeavours and continual assertion of coercive economic and financial strategies over developing nations. China has also been investing heavily in developing regions of the world (i.e., Africa and the BRICS nations) to build their infrastructure. This should help improve living conditions and facilitate these nations to expand their economic capacities while escaping Western mercantilism and predatory loan cycles. (Such as are created by reliance on the IMF and World Bank.) Therefore, although China as a nation is certainly not perfect (with the violent invasion of Tibet being one such example), we see her strengthening influence in international affairs as having a decidedly positive effect on the overall world sphere in the future.

Humans don't think much about how animals want to live. Likewise, the same can be said about China at that time not caring about Tibetan religious attitudes, or its hosts of opinions and beliefs, which made it a loving culture. There is no doubt about this. However, a non-violent being must also bar the eating of animals from his/her life.

What makes our countries proud (i.e., winning the bacon or bread, or promotion of a particular philosophy, religion, or culture) is part of what the Chinese invasion of Tibet was about. Humans develop an attitude (a sense of accomplishment or sensation of delight), as is seen nationally in the Chinese with respect to their invasion. The delight manifests in seeing their achievements manifested irrespective of the pain it may have caused or the environmental destruction. The Chinese found delight in the imposition of their Communistic materialistic attitudes upon the deeply devotional and spiritual Tibetan culture. We have similar attitudes with respect to people's sense of rulership over animals. Thus it is a similar psychological process by which animals are dominated, abused and slaughtered on a massive scale. The justification of the indoctrinated ego on the part of the Chinese is found also in the tendency of meat-eating humans to impose their attitudes upon others. (Via mass advertising and the engendering of prevailing attitudes within the materialistic, avaricious, Western medical fraternity.) We also have the general tendency of countries to psychologically prepare their subjects to define an enemy and thence to wage war (i.e., McCarthyism, or the present promotion of anti-Russian sentiment in the US). The digestion of another country through war and the consumption of meat are similar. Both are obviously brutal and bloody.

One major esoteric reason why Tibet *had* to be invaded is that the monks that should have been *properly* following the *buddhadharma* of harmlessness and lovingkindness to all living things, thus possessing the moral sense to not eat meat, twisted their doctrines to promote meat eating. The unnecessary slaughter of animals thus propagated, and the pain suffered by the animals necessitated that the Tibetan people pay back the reciprocal *karma* they engendered upon a hapless kingdom. Thus were laid the karmic pathways for invasion (consumption) by a ruthless aggressor. There were obviously other causes, such as the violence between warring Tibetan Schools in the past, and the wars promoted in early Tibetan history.

Tibet cannot be properly freed until the monks, following the *buddhadharma* with their hearts, propagate true harmlessness in thought, word, and deed. When they no longer cause suffering (in any inadvertent way) then, and only then, can they reap the benefits of their good deeds. Whilst they are still committing crimes of aggression against another kingdom, how can they hope to not suffer the *karma* therefrom? There is no longer any need whatsoever for Tibetans in exile to continue eating meat products. The vegetarian alternative is now plentiful, especially in India, where the example of vegetarianism is so bountiful in the Hindu religious experience.

The symbology is appropriate, because Buddhism started in India and went to Tibet (including the doctrine of harmlessness). Now that these Buddhists are back in the original home of the Buddha, it is logical that the original methodology for monks be appropriately re-instigated. No longer should animals suffer because Buddhists do not understand the basic tenets of their religion. The *karma* of the Tibetan monks is now especially grave, because many from the West go to them for teachings. Until they can understand this, one of the most essential and forthrightly poignant parts of the *buddhadharma* (i.e., *karuṇā, bodhicitta),* then all the actions and thoughts that flow (the intricate reticulation of *karma)* become the direct karmic burden of the Buddhist monks. They perpetuate much grievous *karma* through their wrongfully conditioned, harmful actions to other kingdoms in Nature. (Thereby they are in fact teaching the doctrine of harm.)

The Chinese were ignorant of the fact that all cultures or differences of opinion should not only be tolerated, but stay untouched, and remain like the prism (preserved as a mechanism of consciousness in terms of a country, creed, or religion). They can only be invaded when the incision is clear (that is, when there are clear and compelling karmic or compassionate reasons). The incision was not clear in terms of China invading Tibet. Neither is it for the animal consumption of present day Tibetans.

The meat eater says: 'I am the human that deserves the subsequent taking of a life, and by extension of this I am warlike. I am the human that once thus fed will be happy'. But here there is a contradiction in terms; such 'happiness' does not take into account the subsequent *karma.* Meat eating and a compassionate religion do not go hand in hand. This is a reason why the atheistic Chinese were so intolerant of religion, and why the Tibetans are so intolerant to advice that they should change their eating habits.

Feeding people's concept of self-identity should not be a factor for meat eating, nor for a country's culture, but Tibetan people religiously continue to eat meat and so suffer the *karma*. Religiously, China continues its regime of killing the spirit of the Tibetan culture, though the worst of such action has now abated. The destruction of life and of lives for one's own gain is sacrilegious. It matters not whether it be the Tibetan culture by the Chinese or the Tibetan's eating of animals. They are both equally aggressive, a non-loving attitude. Why should humans and animals not live harmoniously together, as the rest of Nature does (taking also into account the rightness of natural selection with regards to predatory animals)?

If one is evaluating Tibet and China in the light of this theorem, then one must look at the *karma*. This is why the Tibetan religion is in recess, in terms of its ethics. If one can deduce that Tibet and China are two parts of the whole family of nations, then one is tending to think correctly. One country can do what it is doing because of an open karmic possibility. The instigating *karma* of the harm caused upon animal consciousness by the erroneously applied Buddhism within Tibet is a factor for this, compounded upon by the war-like attitudes of Tibetans in their earlier history. The Tibetan monks should have been the teachers, the exemplars of what is ethically right.

It can be deduced that one country's actions (those of China) are a lot like humanity's in general (with aggressive thinking where no love is apparent). Another country (Tibet) is like an animal (slow thinking, defenceless). No consciousness has the right to interfere with another consciousness without a type of agreement or permission. This has not been given by Tibet to the invading Chinese nor by the animal kingdom to humanity.

To any established religious, or non-vegetarian cultural doctrine, one should ponder the question – why be so cruel? This is what the Tibetan people should think before they eat. Many lives have fallen, have gone into the meat industry, thereby debauching the elegant majesty of the animal kingdom. Many Tibetan lives fell when China invaded Tibet.[2]

---

2   Of course, one could look to the subjective causes for any war scenario between

The law of *karma* is precise; one who causes suffering to another must pay in exactly the amount of suffering caused. It matters little the agent of that *karma,* what matters is that the *karma* be paid back in such a way that the originating perpetuator eventually learns the lesson of what not to do. (Thus one gains a further step on the path to enlightenment, the way of *bodhicitta).* There are interwoven individual, group, national, international, and cosmic streams of *karma.* Thus there are such things as individual diseases, famines, and wars. They are specific effects of the Lords of *karma* bringing the entire cosmic system into one bountiful harmony.

In consideration of all of this, it should be noted that the human body is an animal body or form and must suffer the same type of *karma* as all other animal bodies. Thus, when one eats animal bodies, the *karma* of such action must directly affect the human form. It is inevitable that humans must pay the price of their cruelty – through wars, unloving human relationships, sicknesses, etc. These are often incurred through animal vectors, or the related microscopic members of the animal kingdom (as are bacteria, protozoa, and even viruses). Through sickness and disease much *karma* is resolved. Why cause such *karma* in the first place? It is unavoidable when one consumes the fear and suffering of slaughtered animals. (Certainly, some of such accumulated fear was paid back to the Tibetans when the Chinese invaded.)

What needs to be looked at is the process of war in human psychology; war on the animal kingdom (in terms of meat eating) and war upon the vegetable kingdom through the mass introduction of chemical fertilisers (rather than organic nutrients),[3] causes discordant forms of *prāṇa.* We need to look at how the *karma* works out between one group of beings and those that manipulate them. Human consciousness is elevated from that of the other kingdoms. This is why

---

other nations, or behind the factor of sickness, diseases and the plagues that often beset humanity.

3   One can add chemical pesticides applied on a mass scale to the list. Ultimately here, the problem lies in the present worldwide adoption of monoculture, rather than the ideal of large-scale vegetable gardens that would be found in garden cities. Humanity needs to think organically in order to properly grow their food products, instead of inconsiderate profit-driven farms run by mega Corporations.

we must preserve the harmonious checks and balances in Nature. To work with and to promote the natural harmony of Nature's kingdoms is the responsibility of our greater awareness.

When we look at the internal psychology of the gathering of *prāṇa* or blood (and its rites and rituals), we see that *blood,* particularly in human psychology, has much lore attached to it, and so much meaning. The rites and rituals concerned are patterns derived from hunter and gathering societies. Humanity has now amassed so many forms of ritualised killing that it seems impossible for us not to kill, due to the momentum produced by the blood-letters over the millennia. It almost gives a sense of cultural cohesion to kill, but this must stop if the new era of enlightenment is to awaken. Such a change in behaviour should be initiated by the most sophisticated, aware and advanced societies and religions (such as what Mahāyāna Buddhism represents). If those who are supposed to be the leaders in the ways of compassion are unable to do so, what hope then for the rest of humanity? Yes, the perpetuators of the *buddhadharma* have a moral responsibility to the rest of humanity to be at the forefront of the change away from blood-letting and killing, and not surreptitiously fostering it due to their lack of will to change their habits or mode of thinking concerning the animal kingdom.

To rephrase, over the centuries there has been so much ritual in relation to killing that the related *karma* and thought energy has debased and debilitated human compassion. Of course, the type of magic that strings together *karma* and people's tendencies doesn't help the Tibetan people because their currently established tendency is to kill animals, thus affecting the future cycles or possible expression of that *karma*. One could say that the energy patterns have been laid down for the future, that a ritualised habit has been formed and unevolved thinking is the effect. But this can change if enough people will it so and are prepared to act to produce new *saṃskāras,* based upon active compassion (thus cleansing their former inconsiderate habits).

The mass *karma* and energy of the way people think can be interpreted in seven levels, which from a Buddhist perspective refers to the six Bardo realms and of the way out from the necessity of ceaseless reincarnations. The *karma* of the sum total of the past manifesting through our subtle energy bodies (the etheric, emotional, and mental bodies, and also through all consciousness states), has affected the way people think now. All of the thought and desire impulses from people's emotional minds and desire bodies have stayed in the subjective realms. These thought forms are an indelible force because of the rituals of culturally romanticising all of the killing and slaughter. This romanticised killing has conditioned the masses, making eating meat acceptable. The romanticism involves peer pressure to influence the perception of the way people dress up their meat products for consumption (all the glamour of dining on sumptuous meat dishes). Because of the images formed, people tend to eat more meat. All the desire forms created from all over the world by people to eat meat affect Buddhists (or those of any other culture). They are energised by the ritualised, habitual patterns of the past. Thus one can see why such consumers lay down the lines (i.e., the *karma)* again and again for future cycles.

No matter how sophisticated the rest of one's philosophy or thinking mode may be, condoning meat consumption conditions perpetual repetitious cycles of *karma* producing actions that can lead to birth in hell-like states. The action of perpetuating the suffering of others is simply the bringing down of hell states upon oneself. No 100,000 prostrations, or continuous repetition of the *mantra Oṁ Maṇi Padme Hūṁ,* can possibly save one from self-engendered *karma.* Because the law of *karma* is exact, one gains the good from worthy thoughts of enlightenment and for the compassionate thoughts given to others (i.e., through such devices as *mantras),* but one also must pay for the bad (i.e., *karma* of the slaughter of the animals being consumed). One reaps both the good and the bad, neither can be avoided. The same goes for the Tibetan's that pay for freeing birds in cages in the hope of gaining 'merit'. One gains the good *karma* of releasing the bird, but must also pay for the *karma* of the original trapping and caging of the bird, for its imprisonment and suffering. This goes for whether or not the bird was originally trapped or bred for the purpose of vicarious atonement of the sins of killing, etc. Paying money to the bird-keeper helps keep him alive – 'good *karma'.* The suffering of the caged bird caused by the money exchange process is also the *karma* of the one who pays money – 'bad *karma'.* So the wheel of birth and death turns in the cycle of ignorant actions.

Thus an invocation to any Buddha or Bodhisattva cannot take away what is already there in existence (i.e., the suffering of animals and subsequent effects of *karma*). The thought that the *mantra* can absolve *karma* is preposterous. *(Karma* could not possibly be a law if it is that easily broken.) Buddhists have not properly thought through the effects of *karma*. *Karma* has its own way of making the intended one suffer if the intention is to kill. Killing here naturally concerns the premature death of animals, to eat something that has been killed. Is this not so?

Yes! Buddhists must learn from their own religion and teach compassion in such a way that they are providing positive examples and properly educating others as to the way killing creates *karma*. (It is obvious that the modern sects of Buddhism do not yet understand *karma.)* Humans working out and cleansing their *karma* en masse project Logoi (i.e., all that is) through space towards a fitting conclusion for any *manvantara* (cycle of activity). All things are delineated as *karma* until an appropriate period comes for their cleansing or rectification.

Buddhists must begin to think more globally. By perpetuating certain cultural habits, like the consumption of animals for food, they unknowingly include themselves in arenas of society that promote destruction of the earth and the sentient lives therein. They can no longer separate their meat eating from the effects of the meat industry in the West.

Tibetans may have eaten meat in the past through necessity, because of the isolated steppes of Tibet where crops couldn't produce sufficient yield to support their communities. They, however, would also practice paying respect and honour to the lives sacrificed. This is not the case in Western countries today, where the meat industry is a multi-billion dollar business, slaughtering billions of animals every year. By continuing to eat the flesh of sentient beings (despite being in an environment that caters to vegetarians), the 'supposed' moral teachers that Buddhists represent are surreptitiously condoning the right to commit the atrocities that accompany the mass slaughter of the animal kingdom. By not saying 'no' to this cultural habit, they advertise to Westerners (and even encourage through their living example) that the slaughtering of sentient lives is okay.

Buddhists appear to be ignorant of the effects of the mass rearing of animals in the West, the many cruelties that befall their lives. Shall we visit the slaughter houses and stock yards where these sentient creatures are imprisoned to understand their grief? Shall we see the millions of acres of ancient forests and bio-diversity destroyed for hoofed animals to be bred for meat? The impact of this process goes far beyond the lives of animals. Every life on this planet is affected by such destructive practices.

People must thus begin to understand the terrible impact of meat eating upon the world at large and gradually rectify their behaviour, if the pain and suffering in this world is to eventually lessen. If one proposes religious beliefs pertaining to harmlessness, compassion, and liberation from suffering, then it should not be possible for the proponents to condone the mass-slaughtering of sentient beings that cause no harm to any other being. If one even furtively does so then one no longer upholds virtuous intent. One is perpetuating harm, *not* relieving the suffering of the world (via the uncompassionate 'liberation' of animals through massed butchery).

If you wish to manifest the Bodhisattva vow, you must not be ignorant of the current world issues that cause suffering and pain to sentient beings. Otherwise, how can you uphold your vow to relieve suffering? The Truth of Suffering, and the Truth of the Cause of Suffering are the first two Noble Truths, the foundation of the Buddha's teachings. These Truths should be carefully evaluated in the light of meat eating.

Ignorance is not an excuse in relation to the harm perpetuated. Education on this issue is now manifold. Ignoring it will not save you from the *karma* of killing. The purpose of the *buddhadharma* is to eliminate ignorance in all its manifestations. To turn a blind eye to the suffering of any other sentient being is against the spirit of the Bodhisattva path. Many Buddhists, not truly understanding the way to enlightenment, think that a person can eat meat with impunity and yet somehow be a truely compassionate being (i.e., keeping one's vows of not causing harm to sentient beings). Clearly there is a contradiction here that Buddhism needs to rectify. Sentimental attachments to their eating habits make Buddhists look for excuses to justify their meat eating, in such a way as to absurdly claim that it causes no harm to animals or produces no *karma* of a bad kind. Clearly if one is compassionate, one must think very carefully and correctly on this issue, and simply abstain from the eating of flesh.

Buddhists can no longer insulate themselves on world issues by adhering to parochial forms of consciousnesses. Due to modern mass communications and newspapers, etc., they can readily access information about the problems that affect the world – environmental issues, hunger and poverty, human rights and the capitalisation, globalisation of economies, etc. All such issues relate to the rape of the planet, and cause mass human suffering through the theft of their resources. They are intricately entwined with the production of meat for human consumption. Buddhists must become truly part of the International Community, and set the example of compassion for the world at large. In this task they are currently failing if they continue to condone the mass slaughter of animals.

Let us call to all Buddhists, please begin to lend your hand and give your voice in harmony with those who are so ardently trying to awaken people's minds and hearts to the effects that meat consumption has upon this planet. It is our sincere wish that this short treatise will help to evoke some extended compassion in people, to cease causing harm to all beings by becoming vegetarian, and thereby begin to cleanse the world of the burden of the *karma* of mass slaughter.

Some examples of the destructive effects of the world's meat industry are given in Appendix III at the end of this book.

It can be said that Tibetan people are only thinking in terms of their culture, and in terms of the *karma* of meat slaughter their country is not that bad. (When compared to the way America uses meat products, for example.) Modern processes (unique to the last 200 years), and the changes to the way animals are reared and slaughtered, means that the Tibetans need to reappraise their meat eating. Because Tibetan Buddhists are *giving teachings to the West,* it automatically means they must think more in terms of the sum of the environment they are in. For example, the Tibetan people have moved to Western countries, or to India, and thus must rethink the ethical principle of being a teacher to Westerners (or anyone) they come into contact with.

However, what is actually occurring in this cultural exchange is largely the reverse. The West is teaching the East that it is fine to have multimillionaires and billionaires when the masses are poor and oft starving, instilling in them that avarice in fact is a good and admirable thing in our societies. It promotes the need for meat industries (cruelty factories) and generally indulgent opulent lifestyles. The materialist mentality encourages the wastefulness of planned obsolescence, total misappropriation of the world's resources, and wealth being 'cornered' for the benefit of the relative few rich nations.[4] The general Western mentality has no true love for sentient beings, or of the spiritual processes inherent in and governing all of Nature. Why is the East wholeheartedly taking on board these ideas, and not saying much against them? Why does the East not teach the West that it is not karmically right to be avaricious or to eat meat, nor is it right to condone the environmentally destructive practices associated with these proclivities.

What is lacking in the Tibetan teacher's observations is the scale of the meat industry in the West, and how scale affects everything. It is disgusting the way animals have been cruelly manipulated for our consumer society. It may have been 'correct' for some in the past era to have consumed meat, living in a local environment or scale (as was, for instance, in old Tibet, when there was actually a reverence for the animal life inbred in the population). Such is not the case now in this era of mass consumption and wastage. We expect evolution to proceed in human thinking, as has happened in Buddhism over the millennia, as well as in cultural attitudes. People should have the capability to gradually adapt to higher ideals of psychic purity and compassionate reasoning. We continuously have to shrug off old 'habits' which are no longer useful, whether they be personal or cultural, to allow newer and higher forms of thinking and actions to arise and evolve.

By being the teachers of Westerners, and in condoning the fact that Westerners eat meat, it actually makes these Tibetan teachers directly responsible for the *karma*. You can observe the meat industry and witness all the people who aren't putting up their hands to say no. How unlucky the animals are to have incarnated into a planetary eco-social scheme with humans. Humans are like pigs here, rolling around in the muck of their own habits. Looking at it like this, what makes one any better than the other? (In fact, with this argument the pigs should be preserved and the humans killed, because of the human's actions and

---

4   See, for instance, Noam Chomsky and Marv Waterstone, *Consequences of capitalism: Manufacturing discontent and resistance.* (Haymarket Books, Chicago, 2021.)

'worthiness' concept.) One form of animal nature is *peace-loving*, whilst the other is *aggressive* to its fellow creatures, particularly when all the animals eaten display such harmless qualities. What is also overlooked is the hypocrisy of a nation, such as the U.S. (to take one country as an example out of the many), who on one hand loves animals (as pets) and yet decides that certain other animals should be slain on a mass scale. Why save the dogs and cats from consumption and condemn other creatures to the slaughter? They don't ask to be eaten, therefore if someone does ill-will (some wrong) to them, then that being gets the appropriate action or punishment. In this way, *karma* facilitates the evolution of consciousness.

Conversely, many states in America (a prime meat producer) claim to enact justice today with their 'eye for an eye' mechanism of capital punishment (state sanctioned murder). However, instead of rehabilitating 'criminals', disposing of them in this way demonstrates how little these states actually regard the worthiness of human life.

You have a 'moral' country judging people's merit of whether they should be killed based on whether they are killers or not. The way capital punishment exists in America today is a personification or extension of the way they mindlessly slaughter animals. Once you become desensitised to the slaughter of animals without any sense of conscience, then naturally follows the ruthless conscience-less slaughter of human beings for this or that context. (Such as capital punishment, or engaging in ceaseless wars.) So when we denote that 'the little lamb didn't ask for it' we are simply explaining in our judgement scheme the way we perceive things to be.

Despite their illogicity, the Americans actually have a moral obligation to stop eating meat, based on the reasoning of their present capitalistic justice system. What is in question here is the ideology by which we choose humans or animals to be executed or slain. It is a set of ethics, a moral questioning, or judgement. America particularly elevates its legal system within its constitution, pointing to a need for Americans to have a high code of ethics, morals, and ideals to stand by. However, they have written into their code of ethics that it is alright for the state to kill on the basis of killing a murderer. Therefore, if one is murdering a non-murderer then that one should be deserving of capital punishment (state sanctioned murder). What of the hundreds of millions of murders of animals in that country? Such general hypocrisy, present in most societies today, happens because people have been taught to believe that this killing is needed for their health. Alternatives are not considered, as compassionate thought is absent here. Based upon society's established merits of punishment for murder, where the punishment is death, then animals would not be eaten. However, the problem is that people delineate between humans and animals. But if honesty prevailed, then such harsh punishments for any corpus of sentient beings would not be instigated by those possessing wisdom - *all Life is precious*

The fact that the Americans are not living up to their supposed standards of high morality reveals some major discrepancies in their thinking. The discrepancies apply to moral implications of judgement, and also of their judicial system. The way the judgement is proven barren or 'void of thought' (as a basis of an opinion) has ramifications also for the Buddhists, in that their logic is similarly flawed.

It can be said 'they only hold emotions as their basis of opinion - not cultural mind'. This is preventable by a thorough discourse, thinking to conclusion, examining all of the anomalies and events in history, and analysing the way that wars have been fought over this or that reason. Humanity's advanced thinkers must draw reason from people's aptitude to kill, to find the true motivations there, and to apply it to themselves. They would then find that their thinking here is not sound and that their concept of living up to high moral codes is but wishful thinking.

It can also be said: 'but they think (the important word being 'think') and this is the problem'. However, people 'think' emotionally, selfishly, self-centredly. Thus in capitalistic societies they produce laws aimed at pleasing the little self, based upon such impulses as greed, massive compensation payments for revenge, and revenge killing of those who murdered. If a society can kill humans so easily, then what chance do animals have in their system? With respect to killing, India is in many ways far more moral in their judgements of the worth of animals than the Tibetans and Americans. (Both who pride themselves on being moral.) This is evidenced by India having reverence for the cow, and on the whole will not slaughter it for any reason. India thus still has much to teach the world concerning ethics.

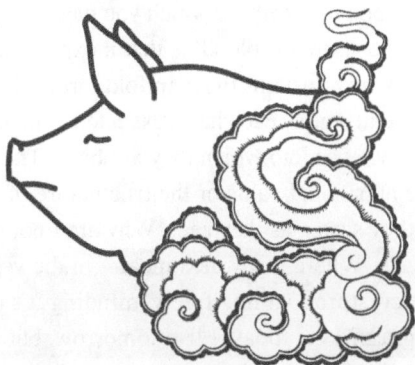

3

The Merchandising of Animals
as Products

An animal in an abattoir has no defensive mechanism when seeing the person in front of it *killing, killing*. At dinner, a person is watching all those around feast on the beast that the eater becomes a part of. The meat industry, served through the purchase of the beast, thinks astutely – *sell, sell*. This is their catch cry to the world community and unthinking 'humanitarians'. They sell to many who supposedly care for Nature (and yet still consume flesh). Let them drink the blood of another to see how the apocalypse of animal suffering tastes!

The argument that 'everyone eats meat' is no longer valid today because of the level of information that abounds about the health benefits of vegetarianism and the harmfulness of consuming animal products. Certainly most of the learned doctors (who are busy 'healing people') do not know about the *karma* of meat, its *prāṇas,* or the effect on health from the consumption of meat. (Indeed, the concept of right nutrition does not fit well in their curriculum at all.) Although *karma* is not explained in our Western societies, it is well known in the East. Surely it is a moral obligation of those in the East, especially Buddhists, to teach Westerners, using skilful means, about the nature of the law of *karma.* It is the blood of others for which you pay your *karma.* A way of looking at this concept of 'blood' is that it expresses the vital Life of an entity, that which sustains the manifold forms of its activities.

People in general simply eat what is expected of them (or proffered to them) by the societies into which they are born. They do not think much about the nutritional value or the true nature of what it is that they eat. Thus they sicken as they age. 'Why am I not healthy?', says one. Another says 'Where is my next meal – in the vegetable patch, or in a sentient creature roaming freely, minding it's own business, quietly eating grass? I eat today, I live tomorrow, but where are my lively locks of gold? Lovely hair gone, to serve the expression of the decay and decomposition that I became as I aged'. 'Why so many aches and pains do I suffer now?' 'Why the loss of function of my organs, limbs or my mind?' 'Why this approaching senility?' 'Why so many doctors must I now face?' I may feel healthy at times, but inevitably I will pay for all this pain and suffering I have caused other fellow animal species - *karma* unleashes itself triply to the subservient. (For one's wrong mental attitudes, the excesses of one's desire body, and through ignorant physical actions.) *Karma* has a way of eating your liver for the one you slay. (An esoteric statement referring to the organ in the body that specifically stores the *saṃskāras* of killing.) You are perhaps a day, a month, or years from dying, but only if you are vegetarian does your diet serve its purpose to free you, free you from much *karma.*

The animal is not yet able to know the way of the heart. But humans, shame on you - 'are you not more evolved than animals?' Then you must pay for what you eat. 'I will consume you in the fires of my belly and see how you like it today. Come what may, I am God and you are not, in that you suffer the *karma* of manifold triple action' the Lord of *karma* says. The wheel (of *karma)* you hold on your head – for all things are an aspect of your consciousness, of the way you perceive things, and your dreams are a reflection of this. So you are trapped in the *saṃskāras* of your own habits. A *saṃsāric*[1] mess is the order today. Clean your body, think correctly and thus compassionately, rid yourself of saṃskāric ways, and your mind will be freed to no longer eat the flesh of other's sufferings. Think rightly concerning the way you behave regarding your fellow humans. Create no more new unfortunate *karma* with them and so cleanse your evil deeds. Also fix up your attitudes to your animal brethren, no matter how strong your desires may be for the attractive packages of flesh provided by the merchants of death. Many cunning lies have been promulgated by the meat industry about the supposed 'necessity' for meat eating. (For instance that vegetables contain no vitamin $B_{12,}$ which they insist is essential for healthy life, etc.) They do not care to inform you of the millions of vegetarians that are healthy and worry not about micromanaging their B_{12} intake. (It is not even a consideration in their lives.) Callous nutritional misinformation serves the purpose of those in the meat industry. They have trapped you into thinking their thoughts are yours and not the other way around. Vegetarians have walked around healthily on the earth for many thousands of years before the indoctrinated attitudes of those that pervert modern scientific theory for their ends. One needs not this modern 'science' (and those that utilise it to merchandise their nefarious products) to be healthy and free in consciousness. Vegetarians simply ate a variety of grains, pulses, vegetables, fruits, and nuts, as they actively went about doing their tasks in life. Through such dietary staples, many disciples of the Buddha and their successors thereby lived long and fruitful lives.

Free the indoctrinators, free yourselves from all such crass attempts to make you the servant of the butcher – eat no more meat. Help the Lords of Life by not having them 'eat you with digestive juices of acid and bile', to consume your flesh to the bone as you sicken and die. (These are karmic strands of two different energy states, major types of *prāṇa* affecting humans.)

In the future, I expect those that do without the meat of others, having paid for former *karma*, to be freed to finally move on to higher enlightened revelation. Theirs is a *saṃskāra*-freed way from compulsive

---

1   *Saṃsāra* is the illusional, fleeting, material world that we all reside in and gain sensorial impressions from.

consumption of meat organs and body bits. They will also free their consciousness from base and egregious mental-emotional attitudes. More refined, closer to divinity, will their *prāṇic* vitality be.

Join yourself to another new view. Love all animals, for they are as you (to be reborn as the next humankind some epochs ahead). In every action you take upon them you indeed kill yourself three times, with your mind, your emotions, and bodily passions. For a human snail travelling through *saṃsāric* time, the causes of *karma* producing action continues on: woe, woe, woe in hell sustaining activity. So free yourself and move faster to a higher enlightened thinking. If you seek to eat the beast, then suffer the kill yourself. You will die someday, and with each breath that you take it will lead to suffering: inevitably you will suffer from those actions of the past. Remember you once were a beast, yet are your motives still bestial now – to slay the cow? Hopefully, you have moved on from where you were several million years ago. You are now human and for that we give you three wishes; abstain from meat, abstain not from peaceful and loving actions, and so to not suffer the throes of *karma*. Rephrased, this could be seen as: abstain from killing, abstain from all pain-engendering karmic activities, and make a new life of the path of Love.

What is being said is that those that do not love animals, who are not kind and compassionate to them, must in fact despise animals. Animal killing is antithetical to the Love that makes one wise and leads to enlightenment. Whether it be a beast, or fellow human, do not kill. All Life is precious, not just what Buddhists call 'precious human life'.

Understand that animals cannot feel the karmic pain you cause upon yourself, as you wet your feet in blood. (The feet symbolise the way that you must walk in life.) Remember the path is long – Love (compassion) in the end always triumphs in the form of the law of *karma,* for *karma* is but the law of compassion in action on a vast universal scale. The long path of Love does not abide in the killing or the will to do evil against the welfare of a person or of animals. There are certain laws for animals and certain laws for humans. Humans live in very complex socio-economic societies and have consciousness, while clearly animals do not. Thus the laws governing human behaviour and the nature of the expression of consciousness are not contained in the animal kingdom. People have to learn to rightly modify and improve their consciousness, to strive for enlightenment and the liberation of all sentient beings, whereas animals simply follow instinctual behaviour. They cannot change or modify their instincts in any way, whereas humans can modify their actions. Therefore, we have a moral obligation to look after animals rightly, not to greedily or mindlessly exploit their innocence, to merchandise their flesh and skin for material benefit.

Did you realise that as a student of *karma* and of the path to enlightenment you must understand the ways animals behave? See, act, and will yourself to be above those who unthinkingly kill one another. It is not the way of progressive human *karma* to follow the nature of an animal in the wild.

No, you must show your capabilities to truly Love, based on a serving attitude to humanity and all life forms. You are not married to the beast, its four-footed nature is not part of you, so why do you effectively make it so by eating it? Realise your evolution has brought you to *look after* the animal by your side so that it is well loved and cared for. If it includes dogs, cats, and guinea pigs, why does it not include a cow? Why should any group of one animal be discriminated against over another group? We should also not discriminate against a person because of the colour of their skin, race or culture. Why discriminate between dogs, cats and cattle? All of you love not the order of being when you intentionally take the life of another. Once your intention is there, they are already dead in your consciousness.

Why kill the animal? Is it because you are unsatisfied in your selfish, sensually demanding life? Do you think it will quench the thirst for life, because you like the taste and stench of the slaughtered, roasted, cooked animal above all else? Try to do better, killing is not the answer. We have enough blood and killing and revenge in wars. Why behave like a crippled malfunctioning society when the war is with yourself? Eventually you will learn not to kill, and so to be more compassionate.

You may be old, firmly entrenched in your Buddhist beliefs, yet you still do not properly understand all the laws of *karma*. When considering human deaths on a huge scale through wars, then this can be correlated to a similar action re the slaughter of animals. Both actions are based on a lack of compassion. Understand that human thought precedes action, causing war, famine, and plagues upon their fellow humans. Move one stage above the folk who are at the level of the instinctual ape-man. Remember that to be a true Buddhist monk (or a Christian, Jew or Muslim), you must never fasten your teeth upon a swine. For your feast is the Buddha's teachings you await: the Lord of Love and energy and all things good. Animals should be cared for, not as meat or flesh, but in the ways of Love. Preserve their lives, resisting staunchly the indoctrinations of the merchants of death.

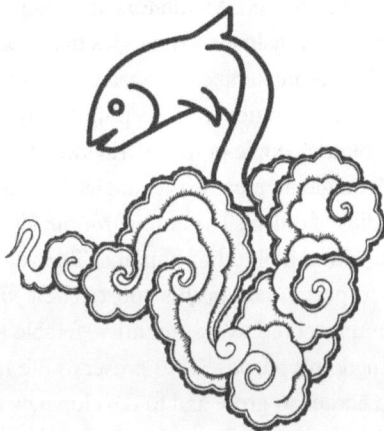

4

The Psychic Perspective

On the realm of mind I see mushroom clouds great and small above the abattoirs, and they trap good thinking people into consuming the matter of meat. Sensible thought does not prevail there. Black magicians play on this feast, syphoning off the *prāṇas* and feeding negative energies through the *nāḍī* systems of the people challenged to not eat meat, and to manipulate others to serve their will. People argue that animal sacrifice is natural upon the altar humanity serves. Little do they know, their children are slowly dying from the consumption of meat. The body can consume only certain amounts of toxic waste. Indeed, the *prāṇas* of decay and death are active in the body of the one eating until the moment of death. Therefore, do not kill other beings and do not eat them, for this assists the activities of the black magicians to sway the thoughts of others upon the subjective realms wherein we live. Little do people think of the existence of this psychic world, but it is certainly real to those with developed inner perceptions. All who meditate aspire to gain high spiritual awareness and transmundane experiences, to inevitably become enlightened. Meditators are attuned to high energy states and are adversely sensitised to energies that produce the dulling of consciousness. We see intolerance to meat eating as a necessary thing to prevent dark or base energies from seeping into the body or mind.

Emotionally volatile people of this world swerve with this thought or that. The black magician meanwhile laughs. He has much fun with the minds and bodies of others. The animal *prāṇic* vitality of meat that he collects flows with the blood of humans. The vegetable kingdom does not, however, participate in this sport. Their *prāṇa* is directly captured sunlight, preserved to sustain all vegetable and animal life. The vegetable kingdom's purpose is to preserve life inside all bodies and to help these bodies to grow and to develop new attributes. Even a cut plant grows again. Its seeds can be dispersed to fill many a field with light. The beast is different, as its legs do not grow back. Humans too suffer forms of *karma* from cutting off such limbs. Nothing can be taken from others without paying an appropriate price. The laws are exact. Nature has exact methods of reproduction, but unaware humanity does not know the effect of the unthinking actions made upon the animal group Soul. Indeed, debts must be paid because the *karma* of bodies is exact. The *karma* is articulate, created by human beings, though *karma* waylays to another time. When coming via the realm of enlightened being the lore is perfect, the law is perfect.

One must also understand the role that *devas* (the angelic kingdom)[1]

---

1   The word *deva* here needs clarification, as the usual trite translation of the term is 'God', or 'gods'. In truth, *devas* represent a whole category of beings that have been thoroughly misunderstood and misrepresented in Buddhist literature. *Devas* constitute such a wide and intricate topic that to properly comprehend it would require an elaborate study too detailed to discuss here. An explanation of their place in the scheme of things is given in my book *The Constitution of Shambhala,* Parts B and C. Each *deva* can be viewed as the sentient Life embodying every atom of matter and category of 'things' in the order of Nature. Their forms are imperceptible by the five senses and the sense perceptors, due to the refined quality of substance they embody. Entities, such as fairies, nature spirits, and the like, up to the greatest *dākinī* (or angel), can all be classified as different categories of *deva*. They make sentience possible in the lesser kingdoms of Nature.

play in the nature of the manifestation of *karma*, for they embody the substance of all that is. *Devas* are conditioned by sounds, either in harmony or out of sync. The energies of meat consumption flowing through the aura causes discordant *deva* emanations. They create aberrant responses in the substance of the human psyche, except in those with low, basic energy fields. Each little *deva* Life (the sentient spirits animating all forms) of the body must be fulfilled with loving energies. Each unit of Life must be rewarded to continue a life unfettered by unwholesome burdens.

The government does not take into account *devas* in the process of governing you, or of any alternative wholesome views concerning health issues. They understand not the subtleties of consciousness fields, or of the intricacies of the law of *karma*. Their onus is the profit motive in all things and so pander to the most profit driven schemes and avaricious people in our societies. For them the meat industry suits the bill. It causes a vast number of unhealthy people from the resultant sickness and diseases through unhealthy diets based upon meat consumption. They crowd into our medical institutions and hospitals, providing gargantuan profits for the pharmaceutical industry and other medical agencies. Part of these profits flow into government coffers, or into the pockets of politicians. For them it is a win-win situation. Massed ignorance is thereby fostered among people about the true situation concerning public health, paid for by the slaughter of billions of animals, and the resultant sicknesses and diseases wrought upon the unwary public.

Devas are very important, affecting all in their embrace. People might think that *devas* don't exist, but they live all around, regardless of what others think. People must begin to see clairvoyantly and to reason appropriately with their minds. We gather information because we *love to learn*. Similarly, *devas live to learn*.

By this is meant that *devas* are fundamentally units of mind/Mind, whereas the quality of *bodhicitta* is technically (esoterically) the guiding force of the human kingdom. Intelligence is feminine in nature and *bodhicitta* masculine. Together they make the dual consciousness-force in the realms of Being. (Thus in Buddhist literature is seen the important place that *ḍākinīs* have in relation to evolved Buddhas and Bodhisattvas.)

The differences between the human and *deva* kingdoms are exact and precise. The energies of your body are internally different – there

are male (human, *piṅgalā)* and female portions *(deva, iḍā),* as in all of
Nature and in the field of consciousness. *Devas* aspire towards greater
light. They sustain what must be and then release their embodiment of
the form when it serves no further use. As they evolve, they liberate
sentient Life from various forms of bondage. (Elemental Lives can also
be trapped in human spawned mental-emotional thought forms). Each
meal is supposed to be a reward to live on, however, the consumption of
meat unfortunately does not keep the integrated *devas* that are your body
appropriately vitalised. They must consequently valiantly try to find the
energies elsewhere to keep your body vitalised and healthy. This is not
too much of a problem when one is young and fully energised by the
Life principle *(jīva)* from the Heart centre. Later on in life though, this
is not the case, and the stored animal and mineral toxins start to assert
their debilitating power on the body, and so sicknesses and various aches
and pains set in.

   Those who are psychic will see the physical manifestation of
sickness in the body as grey, depleted *devas* needing grooming (*prāṇic*
vitality) via more vibrant food. However, when the food one feeds the
devas with is also grey, how can one get internally better? By eating
meat, what is fed to the body inevitably assists the forces of sickness
and disease. This is specially so for high-grade spiritual beings. It may
be hardly noticeable for those whose consciousness is normally dull.
There is thus a natural equation to be found in the balance of life to be
noted. Those whose consciousness state is close to the forms of base
animal vitality will naturally be quite resistant to the adverse effects
of animal *prāṇas,* because these *prāṇas* are of a like kind that they
themselves produce. However, for those spiritual beings, Bodhisattvas,
and astute thinkers, whose energy fields are quite heightened, then the
base animal *prāṇas* produce the debilitating effects noted in this book.

   It makes sense that a dead animal body causes sickness. It is more
than sick – it is dead. That animal has been killed, drained of vital
fluid with the loss of its blood and rapidly decomposes into very toxic
states. Why should one eat what contains the seeds of sickness and
disease? Vegetable matter, on the other hand, retains its vitality for a
considerably longer period of time; for it was intended to vitalise all
animal forms when they consume it.

   What shall we eat? Not me says the Ox, who has died and whose corpse is quickly putrefying in the noonday sun. The matter in the Ox's body is not even healthy enough to keep his body from rapidly decaying, so why should the substance of its decomposition keep yours healthy? Why should you go on eating it to continue to live? It is a slow process, but eventually the food you eat kills you. Not at first, but in the long run. The body is starved of vital fluid *(prāṇa)*, and devitalisation is slow, yet perfectly precise. The universe has its laws relating to the nutritional aspects sustaining the bodily process. So, if you prefer to sustain life, keep eating only healthy *devas* of plant origin. At least these come from devic sources of light. The plant life eats up sunlight and photosynthesis produces its beneficence. Likewise, you must do a similar service by eating the *deva* kingdom in the form of plants, for it is a way that those *devas* can evolve into higher levels of being. Sacrifice is their way to the evolution of Love. Your body is not just your body, it is millions of devic units with their will for you to stay alive, so to love you.

Foster that which is Life. Eat sun energised foods, those foods which have been untainted by humanity's ill will or anti-aphorisms to Love (in conjunction with eating meat). Humans are spiritually more evolved than the animal kingdom, but the majority do not seem to act with the intention to evolve into mature adults. Instead, they act as children of desire and self-serving emotionality. They need to move on and act as if they are in charge. They must act as if they had thoughts of their own, to learn the nature of what is vital and health giving, rather than being buried in the forms of mass ignorance. (The mass-emotions and the psychic currents within which they are caught.)

Only eat clean foods, closest to the fluid vital state of the Buddha-germ *(tathāgatagarbha)* that sustains your life. Your cells are actively seeking the light (just as you must be, if liberated you are to become). How can enlightenment come to those void of light, indeed of the sun's life-sustaining light? The light is the Will. Clean your habits, taste *nirvāṇa*, eat a carrot, watch *devas* play with and energise humans – they love you.

Never fear death, yet do not harbour it in the energy field of your body either, whilst continuing to eat meat facilitates your body's suffering. This is the only way gross energies can be cleansed from the energy fields in your body. Those energies that are coarse and lethargic in nature *(tamasic)* are poured through the *nāḍī* system by the spleen to be finally discharged in a particular organ (via the related *chakra)*. This corresponds to the energy rate most closely aligned to that channel. It is the natural sink or sewer for that energy level. (Energy follows the line of least resistance, or from another perspective – it flows to the weakest point or area in the system). Consequently, in that organ you have a continuous lack of vitality, a weakening of the body's resistance to disease bearing agents. When there is an eventual sickness of the area concerned, gross greyish coloured *prāṇas* are discharged.

Don't eat unhealthy, poisonous, or putrefying things, and all will be fine. Therefore eat vegetables, they are excellent for cleansing out the system with *deva* essences of healthy, captured and converted sunlight, excellent for easy digestion and for easily eliminated waste products. Chlorophyll wasn't made just for plants, for humans can use it too. The *deva* kingdom lives on in numerological coding, in free-flowing energy pathways, and if there are any blocks in those pathways (caused by human action, emotions, or thought), then they will work to remove them, and thus is *karma* cleansed. People who are more inherently psychic will become aware of the free flow of energy, of the love in those that eat not the bodies of our beloved animals.

In time, as civilisation becomes more enlightened, people will think much more of the sentience states of plant life because they will know of the *chakras*. They will be scientifically proven. All of Nature will be seen to contain *chakras*.

Our *chakras* are flowers and our *nāḍī* system can be likened to plants that distribute the vitality or *prāṇic* force to the flowers *(chakras)*.

Therefore, people will come to respect the vegetable kingdom much more than they do now and be totally in tune with the healing potencies therefrom. The science of the solar plant vitality will be well understood and contrasted to the lunar, dull animal variety. It will be obvious which of the two is preferable for human wellbeing, vitality, and good health.

There are further revelations to unfold. See to it you unravel them as you pass through your Bodhisattva training.

Chakras draw on the laws of physics. (One could write a book about the law of physics as applied to *chakras.)* Theirs is a book sealed with seven seals of silence, because its knowledge would be misunderstood by the uninitiated, and therefore tend to mislead and harm those who are untitled (not able) to receive it. Every form in the universe can be viewed in terms of petals of *chakras* (flowers turning as wheels of energies) unfolding.[2] The human kingdom is but one such wheel (the animal kingdom another) and within each major wheel/flower there are countless other flowers (of categories and sub-species). As part of the major wheel, all constituents are geometrically interlinked with energy exchanges flowing from one to the other. In order for the entire system to be wholesome, there must not be a damming up (excess) in any part of the system, or a lack (deficiency) produced in another part of the overall design. If this occurs, then we have a *chakra* displaying abnormal (psychic) responses, or a wilting of the properties of another *chakra* concerned. Many are the lunatics, the psychically insane, psychics, the mad *yogis*, and sickly and hyper-sensitively disposed in our societies suffering from such causes. Put in other terms, there are many of the two major types of diseases occurring (that of inflammation, or congestion of substance).

What then if the major energy circulation between two of the main *chakra* systems on the earth (i.e., the human and the animal) is malfunctioning, with one relentlessly preying upon and vampirising the energies of the other? Is there thus a congestion (excess) of blood *prāṇa* in the one, and a dangerous loss (deficiency) of *prāṇa* in the other? What would one suppose the world's sickness will be as a consequence? How does Mother Nature rectify the imbalance in Herself? The *chakra* system exists in order to produce a healthy body. It is naïve to think that there will be no consequences. Certainly, massive planetary imbalance of *prāṇas* necessitates significant planetary effects for the perpetuators when the *chakra* system reasserts itself to a healthy state. Effect always follows cause, and for humanity this happens upon a mass scale. The bubonic plague, caused by unhealthy living conditions and lice living upon rat vectors, killed much of the world's population centuries ago – a case of the animal kingdom rectifying some of its *karma* with humans. How many times do people need such harsh educational methods of what not to do?

---

2   See my book, *A Treatise on Mind*, Vol. 4, 46.

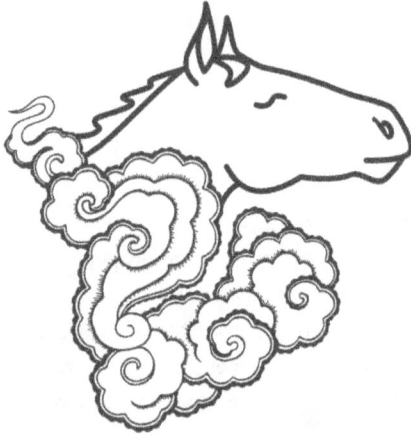

5

The Story of Animal Rebirth

The stories of human beings taking birth into animal bodies abound in Buddhism. Many are found in *The Jātaka Tales*. They are stories purported to have been told by the Buddha, who it was said took such births for the sake of helping sentient beings. The Buddha told stories about people being reborn as animals in order to teach the people simple lessons about goodness to animals and other basic principles of the *dharma*. For instance, there is an example of the sacrificing of Buddha's life to a tigress because the animal was starving. As well as teaching elementary compassion for sentient beings, these examples also taught of the transitoriness of life. Therefore, one should not be attached to the 'possession' of a physical body. There are higher ideals to be aimed for than affiliation to 'self'. The stories intended to stir real devotion to the Buddha and the saints (Arhats). At the time the stories were given, there was also an element or hint of the Bodhisattva virtues that were to be philosophically developed in later Mahāyāna Buddhism.

Of course, if one thought properly about the nature of a 'precious human life', then one can really do much better with it in service to one's fellow beings than to sacrifice it as 'food' to an animal. For instance, one could strive to be a Bodhisattva, or a wise, enlightened being, and consequently help myriads in that life, not just merely one brute animal. (Which incidentally does not have the consciousness to comprehend the nature of the sacrifice anyway.) Sacrifice to animals or taking birth into animal forms is certainly *not* the wisest way to help sentient beings.

For this reason, those initiated into the nature of enlightened being can see that these stories were symbolic (and needed to be so in order to help the consciousness of average humanity at the time), yet they still convey the esoteric truths. They were deliberately constructed in a symbolic way in order to teach the basic values of life to the uninitiated. There is a reason why the Buddha deliberately formulated teachings based on ancient belief patterns. They were 'makeshift' in that they were relative truths that could be reconfigured. Meditative determinations of the way they would affect the consciousness of average humanity well into the future produced such doctrines. They were alternatives, correctly reasoned out, that could give the simple minded an ability to foster the correct understanding as to the way the animal kingdom should be treated.

Since the simpler times of the Buddha, much has changed in human consciousness. Many new ideas have evolved, for instance, entirely new branches of the *buddhadharma,* as well as the entire course of our scientific civilisation. People, en masse, have been taught to receive very complex truths, much more so than 2,500 years ago. Evolution means that the concepts concerned with the making of enlightened beings have also changed. Concepts are therefore being perpetually shaped or upgraded by enlightened Ones who have incarnated for the task. Over time, this process advances the capacity of the human mechanism (i.e., the brain's ability to process information), and thus our ability to think.

The energies of the enlightened mind are therefore of a more rarefied quality than ever before. If one looks to a car engine by analogy, then this can be compared to utilising high-octane fuel upon the human mental and biological processes. The 'car' must make *antaḥkaraṇas* (lines of energy streams) for the qualified energy (petrol –enlightened consciousness) to transform other consciousnesses, or to help them (the other 'cars') move the same way as the Buddha. This energy of enlightenment spreads from one mind to the next, to transform them and so to help them move toward liberation and illumination.

Simpler teachings from earlier times no longer serve the same needs and can now be given with a greater depth of meaning. Some of the 'fuel' that feeds Bodhisattvas has now been put into the pipeline that nourishes the masses of people.

The most esoteric reasoning can still be kept from them, as it is of little value to the student who is an emotional thinker or too dull in consciousness, when clearly the effect of the reasoning is beyond them. A teaching with a simple moral for the people can have several layers of meaning.[1] The literal interpretation is not necessarily the best, and certainly not the most informative, but is intended to be helpful for the 'dull of hearing' (those with commonplace thinking). So how can we try to uplift mass consciousness to new, higher modes of thinking? Or are they forever to remain fixated to the past, and thus not evolve at all?

The necessary outcome of people being kinder to animals could never have taken place if the Buddha had *not said* that you will incarnate into animal bodies. It is a necessary part truth (or subtle avoidance of non necessary details at the time) to convey the true meaning and high ideal of loving animals.

The true or esoteric meaning of what the Buddha was saying is that your physical body is an animal body and it takes the characteristics of what energies you feed it. Eat meat and the physical body becomes psychically the thing eaten, thus you have incarnated into that animal form. This means that when you choose to eat animals, or when you behave in an animalistic way, you embody a similar quality of energy that animals engender – a lower, less evolved form of sentience which your present human consciousness adapts unto itself.

---

1   See my revised book *The Revelation* for more details.

Love the animal kingdom by truly doing no harm, thus not consuming their carcasses, and such animal rebirth will not be possible. Take instead rebirth into the light-filled environment of the vegetable kingdom, by filling the flowers of your *chakras* with the stored enlightening *prāṇas* they contain.

You cannot ask the Buddha what he thinks, but you can approach His temperament if you ask with the right voice. The main reason for the teaching of incarnating into animal bodies is for the right approach to caring and giving to animals, as you would to a child. If you cannot care for this theory, then look at truth for yourself. Little is recorded of doctrines that cannot be deduced to logic. Logic means 'bless the child that reasons that to kill is not the way to Buddhahood'.

Why have the Tibetans found this truth abstracted? They cause death each day for meat consumption. The real issue is - what child can learn nothing from the endearing feature of compassion in Buddhism? If one can but yearn to only love, then the intent to harm is over, guided by the Buddha. One should think about things mindfully and examine the physical implications of one's own actions. This is what the Buddha taught.

What is in question is the way basic doctrines have been consumed by the Tibetans a thousand or more years ago. The teachings given out by the Buddha, whilst being timeless, ageless wisdom, were adapted to the conditions and practices of civilisation *of that time*. When this is not properly understood, there is the danger of dogma that does not adapt the traditional forms of the *dharma* (the body of essentially enlightening teachings and truths) to the *present day* conditioning needs and practices.

The Scriptures concerning rebirth of the human consciousness into animals were mainly for the uninitiated, the unenlightened, those who still needed to learn the overriding import or injunction to Love all things. Thus their need is to learn how to correctly apply the compassionate stance to animals.

This teaching was applied concretely without true thought as to its meaning or purpose, and now we have the repercussions of meat eating in Buddhism, despite the fear of 'animal rebirth'. Today we must move on and properly elaborate what little references we have to the Buddha. We must clarify (and thus initially complicate issues further) because it is part of the esoteric doctrine that must now be given.

Humanity has progressed in the way of intelligence over the last 2,500 years, thus we should no longer be fed by dogmatic teachings that were intended to educate spiritual babies. Let us enrich our lives. The years have left a tide of volatile thoughts and wishes made by the people who haven't understood the doctrine. We need to look to the future, where forging ahead is possible, where we can preserve animals without these silly distortions.

You will come to realise that distortions will be rectified karmically with new knowledge and belief.[2] They are all interrelated in the great wheel of *karma* – within *maṇḍalas* of one thought to another. Cleanse those thoughts as well.

There are serious questions to ask. In this world of busy, intelligent people that has produced the space age and the amalgamation of countries through mass communication, why do the majority of the world's population now eat meat regularly? Why has our technological advancement served such a cruel blow to animals in the fostering of mass propaganda for people to eat more meat? It belies common sense. Animal slaughtering is a multinational affair controlled by relatively few businesses. Yet, by Buddhist logic, this means that meat companies are single-handedly responsible *for all the people that eat meat,* and their consequent *karma.* Likewise, those working with other animal products also take the blow of *karma.* Thereby, in fact, they inadvertently 'revere' these butchers as their saviours, relinquishing their conscience from the need to think any more about the subject. Thoughtlessness indeed is facilitated by effectively thinking that a butcher is akin to a 'Buddha', thus absolving people from their sins.[3]

Regarding the 'absolution of sins': if a meat eating Buddhist's legs were (hypothetically) tied up, intended to be fed to a king at supper

---

2   See my book *Karma and the Rebirth of Consciousness* for detail concerning all of the information regarding animal rebirth presented above.

3   It could be asserted here that the real 'butchers' in this context are the members of the medical profession who do not tell their patients the harm done to their bodies and consciousness through the consumption of poor diets lacking proper nutritional attributes. (They are also unaware of the related debilitating energies.) They are the modern day 'Buddhas' that people and our governing authorities go to for advice on all aspects of health that so much govern people's lives. See my book *Meditation and the Initiation Process* for further information regarding diet.

time, would then the king be cheating *karma* to blame the servant for handing out that meat he consumed, when the king issued the order in the first place? No, it is precisely the king's *karma* and not that of the servant, for the king ordered things thus. It is the same with desire, and it is precisely the same with the meat companies which only serve the societal consumer demand (in modern day terminology), or the vulgar eating habits of people. Why should animals deserve to die for your belly?

The prideful Buddhist presumes that little of the laws of *karma* go unnoticed by him. He laughs first - and meanwhile he chews on an animal's hindquarters, then pretends that the precept of killing permits mantric intonations to annul the otherwise demeritorious or negative consequence of killing.

To put it bluntly, whatever it is purported that the Buddha tells you (probably some later account or interpretation, not direct from the Buddha's mouth, however meritorious it may seem), the fact is that eating meat is demeritorious. (Particularly when the need is not there, i.e., it is not necessary for your health and your survival.) Whatever the Buddhist Scriptures appear to tell you, do not eat the meat of others, or you shall surely owe some *karma* disadvantageous to yourself. One day you may just find yourself experiencing a situation where you are incapacitated in some way, whilst a strangely familiar 'cow' serves you the next details of this equation. It may not be until you find yourself in a hell realm conditioning that you understand what your *karma* forebears.

How far are you truly above the animal kingdom when you create sewers of irrational thought and abattoirs? Are your priests to blame for teaching you? Certainly in Tibetan Buddhism and in our societies in general, the manifest monkey-mind teaching that meat needs to be eaten for every day survival is to be blamed. Indeed, this unevolved mentality explains why industrial livestock activity consumes a quarter of the world's resources.[4] Such irrational thinking is empowered directly by people's emotional desire bodies, which represent the animal portion of their consciousness. (Dogs and cats, for instance, are similarly

4   Symbolically at least, because the real effects, though vast, are hard to quantify. The 'quarter' relates to the physical body's part of the throne of *saṃsāra* – being the dense physical, the etheric, astral and mental bodies.

motivated.) Animal desire directly empowers predatory action upon members of the animal kingdom deemed as prey in order to satisfy an instinct to kill.

Cannot your thinking continue to flourish on higher grounds and avoid stagnation? Do you need a Buddha to tell you in this present age how to think correctly, or are you so meritorious as to prove me wrong? Who are the residents of hell? You won't see me there because I experience the good *karma* and happiness from the lack of pain inflicted upon other sentient beings through my vegetarian diet. Have my words 'unknotted' the saga of your mind, allowing lighted substance to be revealed? Does your meat eating habit cause your rebirth into the animal kingdom, or will sicknesses prevail from life to life? This ignorance (a lack of knowledge of the nature of basic compassion) and 'the immune system *of the world,'⁵* cannot save you, unless you awaken to the true needs of sentient beings.

---

5   The Council of Bodhisattvas, the Spiritual Hierarchy of this planet. They are 'the immune system' because they are responsible for the healing of people's harmful attitudes in life, and of the rectification of humanity's evil imbalances. As do the white blood corpuscles in the body with respect to the invasion of disease bearing agents.

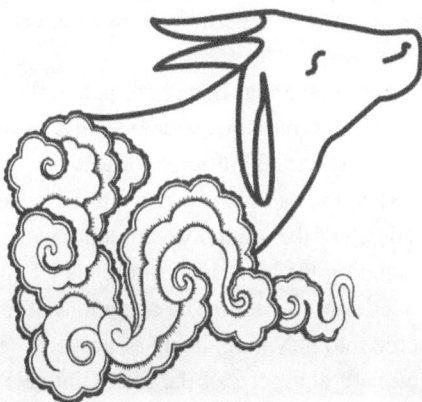

6

Slugs versus Cows

Those desirous of meat often utilise a common defensive ploy. They say:

> 'There's not much point to vegetarianism when one considers the number of insects, slugs, and snails that die in the processes of agriculture. Who can say that any one of those small creatures' lives was less important than that of the cow or pig? So wouldn't it be more compassionate to kill just one cow rather than thousands of insects?'

To eat is to kill, yes, but what sort of sentient beings are you talking about? What lives are you killing and how? What degrees of suffering are you producing and perpetuating? *Karma* is a vast and intricate law, yet it must differentiate finitely. How are pain and suffering reckoned,

according to the dictates of *karma?* Let us say a slug comes along and
eats lettuce that has been sprayed by chemicals and soon after dies.
The suffering here is relatively small. Such death could be avoided too,
if organic foods were grown and the thoughtless use of chemicals in
agriculture was prohibited. Monoculture is the culprit here, whereas
sane biodynamic, organic and permaculture methods would prevent
most such insect deaths.[1]

Irrespective of this, the real issue here is that the suffering of a
vegetable, slug, and a cow, must be measured and compared. They will
thus be seen to be of an entirely different order.

It is not just when the hand comes down upon the slug as it bites.
It is not just the death of the animal we are talking about. The entire
animal's life, including the ecosphere of the planet, are adulterated
due to humanity's desire for flesh. The conditions of modern factory
farming also come into play here, being of perpetual and inhumane
cruelty, where all natural aspects of the life of animals are corrupted
in order to finance greedy profiteers. This reduces many animal lives
to considerable pain, then being disposed of prematurely in an oft cruel
and barbaric way. The animals do not roam in the green fields, hassle
free until their life span is over. Many never even feel the grass beneath
their feet, nor the sun over their head, as in the case of battery-hens.
The entire existence of the animal is being tampered with here, not just
the pain demonstrated at the moment of their death.

Look to the difference of the life span between an insect or slug and
a cow. The life span of a mosquito is reckoned in weeks, while a slug's
is not much longer, but a cow's is twenty years or so. So if you end the
life of a slug prematurely, it may be cutting that life four or five days

---

1   In the search for cleansing vital foodstuffs, organically grown food is superior
to commercial chemicalised foods, but in our consumer societies these are normally
quite expensive. Thus a balance needs to be worked out with respect to one's
finances. If everything else is well thought out, then the body can easily handle
some commercial foodstuffs, for the chemicals are normally eliminated through the
digestive process. Hydroponically grown foods are at the bottom of the *prāṇic* scale,
so should be avoided. There are also food combination rules that should be known
by all who wish for optimal health (see Ayurvedic teachings for more detail). Also,
fasting at times (especially if one feels an illness approaching) is very helpful for
optimal health.

shorter then what it would have otherwise been. Despite its potential for relative longevity, the life of a milking cow in the West rarely lasts longer than five years due to the strain on its entire Life force, whereas a meat cow's life generally will last only one or two years.

Therefore in a comparison between the death of one slug (or even thousands of them) and the life and death of a cow (especially one reared in a factory farm), justice is truly not being served. A cow has a far better capacity to recollect pain inflicted upon it than any slug or insect, and so the *dharma-karma* wheel turns on. Also, the advent of mass-produced animals to fill the myriad supermarket shelves means that it is especially not right to breed the cow and kill it. You induce fear throughout these sentient beings in the form of impure *prāṇas,* and then you consume this fear on your supper table. You may even become angry when someone tells you it is wrong.

The farmer sprays his crop with insecticides and poisons so that the vegetables arrive on your dinner plates without holes in them. But the cows and other higher animals have been killed to provide the leather for your belt or handbag, oil for the soap you use, and many other products, as well as for food.

It is impossible to live without being indirectly responsible for the death of some other beings in some way. This is just another example of the Buddha's First Noble Truth; ordinary existence is suffering and unsatisfactory. When you take this first Truth, in order to try to avoid future suffering for yourself, it is best to try to avoid being directly responsible for killing beings or in any other way accountable for their sufferings. There is a difference between what one consciously chooses to do, and what is unavoidable, and the law of *karma* takes this differentiation into account. *Karma* is determined in terms of conscious volitions for actions in thought, word (emotional projections), or deed.

Whether you are a vegetarian or not, remember that the purification of the mind is the most important thing in Buddhism. The purification of the mind is achieved through overcoming ignorance and attachments to transient things. Now, which is the greater attachment: an aversion to meat, or gross desire for its flavour and aroma? I think that you are fettered by your attachment to meat. The substance of burnt flesh is a very addictive aperitif indeed.

Pigs scream as they are killed. Does a slug do that? A terrified calf rears at the stench of blood and death in its nostrils. A lamb bleats madly as a man applies a knife to its throat. You don't hear the screams of snails, or plants as they die, because there are no throes of their suffering (for they do not have the vertebrate nervous system that allows them to experience this, such as the higher animals possess). Their ability to experience suffering is far smaller, for so too is their sentience. The larger the sentience the greater the capacity to suffer; but the types of suffering change, causing a greater flow of the tears of the Lord of compassion (Avalokiteśvara).

There are injustices, too, of a mass scale upon smaller creatures of the general ecosystem of the planet due to humanity's economic warfare upon it, all for profit. However, the injustice is greatest when considering the mass slaughter of creatures with evolved sentience and nervous systems. The animals consumed have evolved their ability to feel far beyond that of a mosquito. Have you studied them so bleakly as to not notice? Is your thinking so nonchalant concerning the teachings of the Six Realms[2] that you have forgotten about the existence of the hell realms, where the *karma* thereto is related to your motive for killing, and the amount of suffering you actually *do* cause when you do so?

One must learn to properly count, not simply with one's desire mind racing, but with a placid, more aware, loving mind. One slug simply does not add up to one cow. The sentient lives killed in the production of vegetables are of an entirely different level in their ability to experience pain than what is experienced by higher animals. One could even argue as to whether or not these lower sentient lives experience any pain at all. It is a moot point for plants or insects, but not so for the higher species of animals that humans consume in vast numbers.

The *size of the animal* is also an important consideration. A cow contains billions of cells, an insect consists of only a tiny fraction of this. It would require millions of mosquitoes to constitute the bulk matter of a cow, yet this amount of mosquitoes does not add up to the awareness level of one cow.

---

2   See my book *An Esoteric Exposition of the Bardo Thödol,* Part A for an explanation of these.

Millions of cells in your body die daily, but still those millions of dying cells do not add up to one human being, similarly with smaller life forms, such as insects. Millions of lesser evolved sentient entities do not add up to the awareness state of one far more greatly evolved animal. The evolution of consciousness is progressive; it is about quality rather than quantity.

If one does not count the size of things properly, then one is ignoring what life is all about. Does the life of one atom equal the life of a planet? Does the life of one cell equal the life of a human being? By the same token, how can the life of one slug (or many slugs for that matter) equal the life of one cow, a far more complicated organism? Slugs and insects have been designed by Nature to evolve in large numbers and to die in large numbers with only a very few surviving to produce the next generation. That is how the economy of Nature and the evolution of species works.

This is not so with cows or the higher forms of animal life. Only humanity has created an imbalance in Nature by deciding to prey on select types of animals specifically for their various forms of blood rites.[3] Blood is the essence of higher sentient life, therefore the spilling of blood is what *karma* is mostly concerned with, because 'blood is Life'. This is an esoteric fact not understood by those with dull comprehension. Insects do not have blood. Blood necessitates a heart to pump it and a heart is relegated to higher sentient beings. Being concerned with the heart of things signifies the beginning of the development of the quality called Love.

Please learn to count with a little insight into the nature of 'Life' and its manifold vehicles, to see that one slug simply does not add up to one cow. To assert such an equation only shows a lack of clear thinking in relation to the life of animals, and is concocted up as an absurd justification for meat eating by the ignorant.

It is plain to see that the consciousness level of a cow is far raised beyond that of a snail. Cows, pigs, and sheep all have nervous systems (externalised correspondences to the *nāḍī* system) with a certain number of *chakras,* and thus a greater level of sentience. This is important as it

---

3   The reference here is also to forms of animal sacrifice performed in many religions throughout the ages.

equates to the degree of suffering experienced by that life, and suffering is what we are trying to transcend, is it not? Thus let us truly understand suffering in all its subtleties in order to unchain sentient beings from it.

We agree that all Life inevitably produces suffering, that death is inevitable (and even liberating), and that every time we breathe we kill. Let us not be incompetent thinkers (when clearly we are capable of realising with the use of our compassionate reasoning) to espouse that the life and death of a cow is no different to that of a slug.

Incompetent thinking it certainly is, to compare swatting a mosquito with the slaughter of a cow. Are you telling me that you see no difference in this? How can one equate the death of short-lived insects with the gross cruelty and imprisonment of animals, culminating in slaughter of these, our grossly ill treated fellow sentient beings. They are in fact our brothers to be, humans in the future. Why present shallow justifications and explanations to condone the cruelty perpetuated upon animals so that meat can be consumed?

There are things you can avoid killing and there are things you cannot. Thus the quality of the life being killed is important. If the Buddhist concept of rebirth is feasible, then, is that cow or insect a human being? Why kill either? It is unavoidable in the case of insects (like that of the cells in your body), but the killing of cows, sheep, etc., is clearly avoidable. The cow has come far further than insects, it is closer to a human in consciousness (closer to the development of mind).

In a similar way to humans, insects such as bees and ants have developed a more sentient social structure. The life of one worker bee does not matter greatly to the existence of the hive as a whole. The single bee has a limited life span, but to it the hive is all-important. It sacrifices its life for the welfare of the hive – thus it will sting you and die if necessary. Higher forms of animal life have a far greater sense of emotion and feeling then their less developed animal counterparts. There is a problem in the lack of understanding of the way evolution unfolds, thus the true teachings on rebirth have been confused. Is it so hard to understand that a pig is in fact more evolved than an insect? It is more human like, and if you do not see humans as being more developed then animals (beyond the factor of positive rebirth, good *karma*) then what is your reason for not eating humans as well? What is your reason for not taking advantage of road kills and elderly deceased? Surely by your logic this would be a more compassionate act than killing something to eat? Is it catching diseases from such corpses you fear? But are not dead animals equally corpses? Surely human flesh could keep your body and mind strong, just like the animal flesh you claim to need for such reasons.

It's a shame that many (being too desirous of meat) don't care to know about the numerous diseases animal consumption actually causes. Inevitably, meat consumption only makes your body and mind weaker and weaker until sickness prevails. Death is inevitable, but you make it ever more painful with your will to kill.[4]

To purify your mind is to reason without desire. Only desire, not rationality, allows one to conclude the absurd, disproportionate equation that it is preferable to kill larger, more advanced animals than insects and slugs.

The desire for meat in many is strong. Without it they may be able to reason with Love and understand what *bodhicitta* really is. You who choose meat do not comprehend the nature of *bodhicitta* because, by your circumspect reasoning, you do not understand that the way of release from suffering of all sentient beings happens in accordance with the way Nature intended.

One tries to preserve life, and refrains from killing to the best of one's ability. This of course does not mean being over zealous in the aversion to causing death. Some of which are naturally unavoidable (i.e., by the time we take a new breath we may have killed millions of micro-organisms too small for our eyes to register).

The fact of death is unavoidable, and we can only compassionately try our best *not* to kill. But Buddhists must begin to contemplate the hierarchy of sentience and the multifarious, varying levels of consciousness housed in such forms. All Life can be contemplated in terms of suffering, but not all lives suffer in the same way or to the same extent.

As Buddhists are trying to transcend suffering, it is best to produce as little *karma* of killing as possible. Such killing *saṃskāras* do prevail on to the next life, and bring with them the suffering that was inflicted

---

4   This subject has already been dealt with above.

upon other sentient beings in previous lives. This is especially so for those larger forms of animal life which have the greatest capacity to feel, and thus to suffer.

Five fingers do not make a hand, unless those fingers are attached to the palm, and the palm to an arm, and the arm to the rest of the body. Neither do thousands of slugs make a cow, even if the sum total of their weight equalled it in bulk. They are, however, part of an ecological order, a hierarchy in Nature that places cows and larger animals near the top of the list of animals because of their more evolved nature, and slugs, snails, and insects near the bottom.

Those at the bottom of the list breed in the billions or trillions, where those at the top breed in thousands. Those at the bottom are of small size and comparative sentience, and those at the top of greater size and sentiency. For each natural death of the one at the top, millions of those at the bottom will have died and may be reborn several, if not hundreds of times.

Life thus goes on. It is consequently not possible to justifiably suggest that the life of an animal at the top of Nature's hierarchical list be equal to a sentient entity at the bottom. The same goes for the hierarchical lives that go into the constituency of a human being. One can rightfully kill a cell or a grouping of cells in the body (each cell being a unit of sentience), especially if those cells are diseased. However, to kill an organ (which is near the top of the human bodily hierarchical organizational structure) would be dangerous for the well-being and viability of the body as a whole. The scale or size of what is in consideration does matter.

If Buddhists do not take the scale of things into account, and also the quality of sentience, then they might as well say that the life of one cell in the human body equals the life of the entire body. People do not normally go about consciously killing the cells in their body, but this is what happens millions of times each day through the process of normal living. By the argument given above, that the life of a slug is equal to the life of a cow, then this cellular slaughter would translate as being the same as killing millions of people.

Another point to this argument is that because the natural tendency of slugs and snails and other insects is to breed in massive numbers and eat only vegetables, vegetables necessarily have some defences against them. There are also a host of allies to the vegetables (such as birds, humans, and other insects) to help in their defence, so that pests do *not* get the upper hand in consuming the vegetable kingdom, as *all animals* need to live upon vegetables in one form or another.

Even carnivorous animals eat the animals that feed upon the vegetables. These carnivores have no choice in such killing, but humans have a choice, and this is the point. Another point worth mentioning is that humans *must* kill the predators and pests that would threaten their survival on this planet. Species that threaten to kill crops that humans need are inevitably the slugs, snails, and insect pests. (If their numbers were not rightfully reduced by the means that Nature has devised.) In this humans have no choice, any more than having a choice in killing disease bearing organisms (such as bacteria) that threaten their lives. We can thus state (unequivocally) that it is an essentially compassionate act to *wisely* kill the slugs and snails that threaten the lives of all plant eating species. But this is not so for higher order animals. We do not need to, and certainly should not, breed them for slaughter (any more than we need to breed slugs and snails for slaughter). We simply need to rightfully control the population explosion that would occur if no checks were made to ensure that they do not get an upper hand in the biosphere.

Thus there is a choice in the killing of higher forms of animals that do not threaten the life of everything upon this planet, if they were left to their own devices in a natural environment according to the way Nature designed things to be. Humans have destroyed the natural balance of Nature, thereby causing massive insect plagues, and greedily (for monetary gain) breed animals so that they can be slaughtered as a commodity of exchange. There is no Love here for the true value of Life, no compassion for the suffering of their animal brothers. The creation of unnecessary blood letting is out of carnal desire for the offering of carcasses to the mammon that belies the graveyards of their bellies.

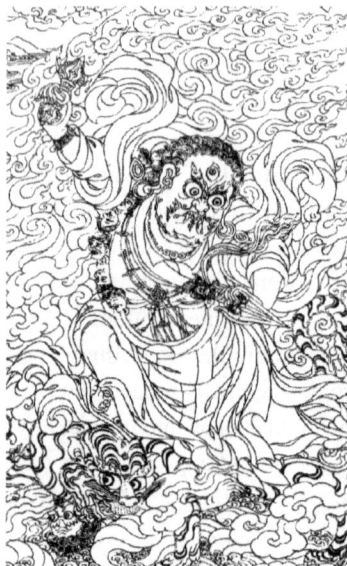

7

The Highest Yoga Tantra

Or:

**It is all right to eat meat because
I think I am like a great *yogi*
living in the Himalayan snows.**

In this section I shall endeavour to answer many of the assertions of those that claim they are actually practitioners of the white (Buddha) *dharma* whilst they eat meat. There are a potpourri of reasons why Buddhists of various orders have convinced themselves (and others) that this form of addiction to *saṃsāric* pleasure does not forgo the Buddha's strict guidelines as to the only way that one can get away with the eating of meat, so that they would not immediately be cast out of the *saṅgha* during his time.

The only recorded time when it is purported that Buddha ate meat whilst being Buddha was when it killed him.[1] The *saṃskāra*-laden individuals and groupings that call themselves Buddhists should meditate deeply as to what this, the last great act of the Buddha, is *supposed* to teach humanity. Namely, do not kill, even surreptitiously by eating meat; it will destroy the awakening Buddha within you. It kills, it poisons, it is a gross act of *adharma,* an ignorant folly that does no good to any being. Why cannot Buddhists understand this, one of the most basic, simple, dramatic and poignant of the Buddha's teachings, requiring no great wisdom to comprehend? Even those with mean or little intellects[2] should understand this. If they cannot, what then do they understand of the *buddhadharma?* The question posed simply is: 'what is it that can kill a Buddha?' The answer: eating meat. They should ask themselves as to why the Buddha (undoubtedly the wisest and most enlightened of all beings to teach humanity in recorded times), chose this as his last major teaching. He utilised whatever bit of *karma* he had left[3] with the material world via eating the 'pig meat' as a mechanism to gain his *parinirvāṇa.*

One of the reasons why pig meat was chosen to play such a prominent role is that a pig is considered to symbolise the filth, murk, and most foul, disgusting mire of *saṃsāra,* from whence it derives its sustenance. Whatever enters the bodily system and is digested becomes *prāṇa* that must be circulated in the *nāḍī* system. So what is it in reality that made the Buddha sicken and die as a consequence of eating (symbolically rather than effectively[4]) this pig meat? The answer is plainly evident

---

1   This teaching from the *Mahāparinirvāṇa Sūtra* was quoted earlier.

2   They are the lowest of the three categories of listeners of the *dharma.* The average listener (those with 'ordinary intellects' being able to properly understand conventional truths), whilst those with superior intellects being able to gain an understanding of the nature of absolute truth.

3   Omitting the polemics here as to whether the Buddha actually had any *karma* to express.

4   Below is a quote from Chapter Eight of Suzuki's translation of *The Laṅkāvatāra Sūtra,* which points out that the Buddha definitely could not have partaken of flesh of any form at any time, even before his death. (Translated from the original Sanskrit by

to any who want to rationally look at the symbolism – the most foul, filthy, disgusting type of *prāṇa* which even the Buddha's immaculately radiant *nāḍī* system could not properly transmute at that time. If the Buddha is purported to have not been able to transmute such gross base energy, then how much less can a mere aspirant on the path? This was the direct teaching given to us by this final act of sacrifice.

Note that a pig is depicted as one of the three animals in the centre of the Wheel of Life, symbolising the darkness of ignorance and of ego-delusion.[5] It is the blind energy of groping in the mud and mire of *saṃsāra* that keeps people bound perpetually to the wheel of birth and death.

How can one put into the 'difficult-to-obtain, free, and endowed human body'[6] the most base *prāṇas* and still think of it as preciously endowed? How, therefore, can those purporting to follow the Highest Yoga Tantra free themselves from the blood of the suffering ones they fill their *nāḍī* systems with? They claim that by some great, inconceivable reason, they are somehow learning the art of detachment this way. Detachment from what, one can quickly question? All that can really be seen is their attachment to conventional thinking and rigid, unyielding devotion to the social mores of the society they were born into.

Rather, they should be as Avalokiteśvara , looking down from great heights, crying tears of compassion for the suffering of all sentient beings and vowing to never cease striving until those suffering ones

Daisetz Suzuki. Routledge & Kegan Paul Ltd. 1932, 1973.) See Appendix One for the major portion of the translation.

There may be some, Mahāmati, who would say that meat was eaten by the Tathagata thinking this would eliminate him. Such dull witted people as these, Mahāmati, will follow the evil course of their own *karma*-hindrance, and will fall into such regions where long nights are passed without profit and without happiness. Mahāmati, the noble Shrāvakas do not eat the food taken properly by [ordinary] men, how much less the food of flesh and blood, which is altogether improper. Mahāmati, the food for my Shrāvakas, Pratyekabuddhas, and Bodhisattvas is the Dharma and not flesh food; how much more the Tathagata! The Tathagata is the Dharmakāya, Mahāmati; he abides in the Dharma as food; his is not a body feeding on flesh; he does not abide in any flesh food.

5   The other two animals are the snake, representing anger, and the cock, representing attachment.

6   From W.Y. Evans-Wentz, 'The Precepts of the Gurus', page 67 of: *Tibetan Yoga and Secret Doctrines* (Oxford University Press. 1958. 1982).

have been relieved from their suffering. One cannot do so whilst the belly resonates a lack of true ethical morality and compassion because of attachment to gross *prāṇic* states. How can eating animals relieve them of their suffering, when they have been butchered to satiate an addiction to meat? How can meat eating Buddhists earnestly chant the *mantra* of Chenrizig; *Oṁ Maṇi Padme Hūṁ!* (or any other *mantra* for the relief of suffering of sentient beings) and not be a hypocrite in their utterings? How can they thereby act as advocates of the Buddha *dharma* if they do not even emulate the Lord of Compassion with sincerity?

They will not free themselves from the shackles of mind-borne *saṃskāras,* nor from the *karma* of the massed suffering they have caused. Yet they were supposed to be the teachers of the younger ones on the path (as supposed exponents of the *'highest'* Yoga Tantras). The *karma* of those they have misguided has fallen on their shoulders because they should have explained the truth concerning the nature of their addictions, and not the masquerade that they demonstrate. Although they may gain some good *karma* if they earnestly intone *mantras* for the relief of suffering or for the release of those they have helped slaughter (it may even help them to be born as vegetarians the next life), inevitably they will have to pay the *karma* of their evil doing. They will receive the effects of both streams of *karma,* for that is the only way this law can manifest and still remain a law.[7]

Now to answer people's projections concerning the greatest of the sages of past times (such as Tilopa, Milarepa, etc.), of those that lived in the charnel places, cemeteries (and the like), who were purported to eat meat. (The reasoning being presented is that because these great sages could do it then, so can we now.) Modern teachers, living in the comforts of their monasteries (and the like), having nowhere near the true spiritual heritage of the sages (i.e., their level of attained Bodhisattva *bhūmis*[8]) may only pretend to be such accomplished *yogis*. The great ones utilised seemingly minor infringements of the (good) Law, chosen as modes of

7   The nature of the law of *karma* is so misunderstood that my book *Karma and the Rebirth of Consciousness* will try to correct the misinterpretations and illogic that abounds regarding this subject.

8   This, of course, is presently debatable for most 'gurus' because of the titles accorded to them, but can be proven, once the mechanism for such perception has been accorded to those who would wish to ascertain the truth.

education for their most accomplished students. Although this practice may have been applicable in the past ages, such is not possible now. The entire world must now be rightly educated as what not to do (such as to not eat the results of the butchery of millions of animals each year). This is what *must* be taught by the compassionate. There is a most pressing need to rightly educate, which the true Bodhisattva *must* heed. The worldwide scourge of the killing of animals is a horrific and unending pandemic, for which no great one can watch without great compassion. Nor can they partake any longer in a share of the rivers of blood shed every day for the sake of the world's addiction to this form of thinking.

Let us look to the symbolism, to the lifestyles of the *yogis*, as to what they had to accomplish relative to their time. Their concern was the nature of the required shifts in consciousness needed to eliminate the subtlest forms of attachment, which at that time was to the development of compassionate action.

A good example is the life of Milarepa. He practiced extreme asceticism, and it is stated in his biography that after living for a long time on only nettles (giving his bodily complexion a greenish pallor), some hunters came upon him and left him with the remainder of their provisions and a large quantity of meat:

> saying respectfully, 'It is praiseworthy of thee to practice such asceticism. Please pray for the absolution of the animals we have killed, and for our own sins in killing them.'
>
> 'I rejoiced at the prospect of having food such as ordinary human beings eat, and, on partaking the food, I enjoyed a sense of bodily ease and comfort, and a cheerfulness of mind which tended to increase the zeal of my devotional exercises; and I experienced keen spiritual happiness such as transcended anything I had known before....[9]

He ate this meat very sparingly until maggots appeared upon it and then stopped all together in order to allow the maggots their feast. Later, he was offered: 'some well-cured and seasoned meat and butter, and a goodly supply of *chhang* and flour'.[10] The text then states:

9   W.Y. Evans-Wentz, *Tibet's Great Yogī Milarepa*, (Oxford University Press. 1928, 1969), 199.

10   Ibid., 205.

On my partaking of the good food, my physical pains and my mental disturbance increased so much that I was unable to go on with my meditation. In this predicament, thinking that there could not be a greater danger than the inability to continue my meditation, I opened the scroll given to me by my *Guru*. I found it to contain the manner of treating the present ailment, thus clearing the obstacles and dangers to the Path, and turning the Vice to Virtue, and increasing the Spiritual Earnestness and Energy. It was mentioned in the scroll that I should use good wholesome food at this time. The perseverance with which I had meditated had prepared my nerves for an internal change in the whole nervous system, but this had been retarded by the poor quality of my food. Peta's *chhang* had somewhat excited the nerves, and Zesay's offerings had fully affected them. I now understood what was happening.....The practices then conferred to him 'the power of transforming myself into any shape [desired], and of flying through the air...[11]

We know that *yogis* in Tibet were caught in a trap, or conundrum, where because of the high altitude and harsh climate, there was little to eat except ground barley, dairy products, and meat. To stay alive, the people had to eat meat. The *yogis* therefore had to develop ways of transmuting the worst effects of the meat consumption. The quotes extracted from Rechungpa's biography of Milarepa nevertheless prove illuminating. First, he comes out of a major period of meditation, of being breatharian at times, and at other times manifesting a form of extreme veganism; living upon a mono diet of relatively non nutritious nettles. The release of *prāṇas* obtained from eating a more nutritious diet (of meat) gave him the experience of 'keen spiritual happiness such as transcended anything I had known before'. When this statement is read esoterically, in accordance with the way that Tantras should be read, we see that what was fully awakened in him were the *siddhis*[12] associated with the Solar Plexus centre *(maṇipūra chakra),* which confers 'spiritual happiness', being the emotive centre in the body. It is also the *chakra* that synthesises all animal *prāṇas* in the body, as will be explained in Volume 2 of my *A Treatise on Mind* series.[13] This

11 Ibid., 208-11.

12 Psychic powers.

13 *Considerations of Mind: A Buddhist Enquiry,* 28.

then was the high level of his yogic development, wherein the eating of meat toxins was possible in order to gain revelatory experiences.

His meditative unfoldment necessitated a progression from the full awakening of the *maṇipūra chakra* to that of the Heart centre (the *anāhata chakra),* from whence is derived *bodhicitta.* In relation to this development, we are told that the next time that he was offered 'some well-cured and seasoned meat and butter, and a goodly supply of *chhang* and flour', he found that 'On my partaking of the good food, my physical pains and my mental disturbance increased so much that I was unable to go on with my meditation'. So what happened to him? Tantrically, the answer is simple: the Heart centre is the *chakra* in the body that deals with *prāṇas* innate within the human kingdom concerned with the generation of *bodhicitta.* Animal toxins are not in any way compatible with the force of compassion (being in fact antithetical to this force), thus he suffered the negative effect of the meat toxins and the Chhang (a type of beer). What was the cure to his suffering? The answer was given on the scroll offered by his guru to be read at this time (the most dangerous period of his meditative career). He had to obtain 'good wholesome food at this time'. If the food containing meat was termed 'good food', then 'good wholesome food' concerns the consumption of food that contained no meat, thus making it 'wholesome' – able to properly generate *bodhicitta* and all of the ramifications that the resultant full enlightenment bestowed. It is the way of the Heart centre (not the *maṇipūra chakra)* that allows the experience of *śūnyatā.*[14] The way of the Heart necessitates the full awakening of *bodhicitta,* hence the impossibility of the intake of meat toxins at this stage.

Nowadays, it is not necessary for practitioners of the yoga Tantras to suffer as Milarepa did. Their entire meditative progress can be quickened through eating 'good wholesome food' right from the start. Indeed, this *must* be so, as the need for proper compassion to the animal kingdom is overwhelmingly great in this modern era.

It should be noted that all great *yogis* (such as Milarepa, who had to eat meat because of the environment in Tibet in which he lived) have

---

14   The Void, the nature of the liberation attained when one has successfully traversed to the 'other shore' from *saṃsāra.*

had to take rebirth again in order to cleanse the 'evil doing' of the toxins they have ingested. This is needed to cleanse the karmic residue of the animals they have helped kill. This is the law, and no great one is truly liberated without such cleansing. The *karma* persists and persists. Thus they remain Bodhisattvas (and do not become Buddhas) until this *karma* is cleansed through right (educative) action in a later life. In Tibet, they had developed the *siddhis* to transmute the gross effects of the meat *prāṇas*. (Meat being relegated to the physical realm after all, whilst the *yogis* attained potent energisations from far higher realms of realisation.)

What was needed out of necessity by great *yogis* in the past cannot be mimicked by modern exponents of the yoga systems, *as if* the conditionings that the great ones had to bear are still with us. They are not (and never again will be with *yogis*). Modern mass communications and transport systems have seen to that. In the world today, all types of food can be sent relatively easily to any place of the globe at need, even Tibet. The Council of Bodhisattvas now take the full interpretation of being compassionate to the whole world as a major teaching for humanity to follow. It cannot be any other way; people are no longer handicapped by the physical hardships of ancient windswept Tibet, and the indigenous meat consuming society through which they *had* to project their accomplishments. (Despite the meat consumption and *not* because of it.)

All of the stories concerning the great *yogis* and *mahāsiddhas*[15] of the past are Tantric texts, and accordingly must be rightly interpreted ('unknotted'). Tilopa is a case at hand, where the fact that he often appeared as a fisherman is quoted. This, however, was but a *conjuration* of a bodily manifestation for the purpose of rightly educating 'sinners', as stated:

> He [Tilopa] took other bodily manifestations and explained the Dharma
> to sinners. He showed himself in innumerable ways: as an artisan, as
> a great meditating siddha, as a fisherman, as a hunter, and so forth'.[16]

---

15 Great accomplished ones, who have attained all of the powers through meditation that enlightenment brings.

16 Vyvyan Cayley (Ed.). *The Life of the Mahāsiddha Tilopa* (Library of Tibetan Works and Archives. 1995), 54-5.

The fish may have been Tilopa's symbol, but nobody knows whether or not he was actually a fisherman.[17] Likewise, it is unknown whether or not he caused fish to appear magically (especially as his body was a magical conjuration) as Jesus did when he fed the five thousand gathered to hear him with a few fish and loaves of bread offered to him by a boy. The fish symbolises discipleship, as all are swimming in the (emotional[18]) Waters of *saṃsāra*. Depending upon the size of the fish, so we have the nature of the spiritual age of the disciple caught. This is one reason why Jesus asked his disciples to follow him, so that he could make them 'fishers of men'. Until people can read esoterically (and thus properly decode the statements made by the great ones in terms of the language of the enlightened), they should reserve comments concerning the stories of the *mahāsiddhis* to themselves.

A line of reason that is often given by (supposed) followers of the Vajrayāna is similar to that stated below:

> The Tantric path or Vajrayāna has four classes. In the lower classes, external cleanliness and purity are emphasized as a technique for the practitioner to generate internal purity of mind. Therefore, these practitioners do not eat meat, which is regarded as impure. On the other hand, in the highest yoga Tantra, on the basis of detachment and (compassion), a qualified practitioner does meditation on the subtle nervous system, and for this, one's bodily elements need to be very strong. Thus, meat is recommended for such a person. Also, this class of Tantra stresses the transformation of ordinary objects through meditation on selflessness. Such a practitioner, by virtue of his/her profound meditation, is not greedily eating meat for his/her own pleasure.
>
> Upon answering questions regarding vegetarianism, Tibetan Buddhist's will often respond that it is the lower path to follow the strict disciplines of vegetarianism.

One should note that the Vajrayāna path (the path of Tantra) is said to sit as an apex above the two other paths (the Hīnayāna and Mahāyāna),

---

17 The symbolism can well be as that provided by Jesus when he said: 'Come ye after me, and I will make you to become fishers of men', *Mark 1:17*.

18 The emotions or the emotional-mind, which is where most people are centred, is governed by the Watery Element, as the emotions are fluid, turbulent, etc., like water.

and is said to be the fastest, most direct way of attaining enlightenment. The view of the Vajrayāna is that all things in the phenomenal world have the potential to lead us to enlightenment. Thus it attempts to utilise the sacredness of all experiences as the most direct method to realisation, the attainment of *śūnyatā* and enlightenment.

Do the normal interpreters of this doctrine mean to say that the followers of the Vajrayāna are above the law of compassion (i.e., do not need at all to be loving or compassionate)? No! The only ones that follow Tantra and are non-compassionate are members of the dark brotherhood (i.e., sorcerers and the like). What can be derived from our understanding of the above quotation is one (or a combination) of three things:

1. If in the path of Tantra, passions and attachments are said to be used as a mechanism to reach the state of emptiness, then what we are really looking at are elements of the black Tantras that have vicariously found their way into the true white *dharma* over the millennia, and should be eliminated.

2. The practitioners have not understood the symbolism associated, for such texts involve the highest amount of coding by enlightened beings to ensure complete safety from readers prematurely developing *siddhis*. The exponents of all teachings are karmically responsible for the effect of their teachings. The enlightened ones certainly knew this when they encoded 'ear whispered truths' in such a way that only those properly initiated (by a truly enlightened sage) could understand. Where does one find such a fully enlightened and universally acknowledged sage today? In Vajrayāna, there is said to be a method for transforming attachment into the path, but to practice that method one must be very skilful. This skill entails having one's attachment become the cause of experiencing great bliss and then using the mind of that great bliss to meditate upon emptiness. This may be the theory, but the means of the practice is something little understood by anyone other than s/he who is truly enlightened. Of course, one can look to such 'skilful means' (as exemplified by Marpa's teaching to Milarepa given above), but it has already been stated that this was only for extreme cases, and cannot be applied truthfully in conditionings existing today.

3. An erroneous doctrine masquerading as a Buddhist text written
   by someone (a black Tantrist) claiming to be someone else (i.e., a
   great sage). Somehow through the mists of time that text has been
   accepted as the writings of the sage.

This is not the place to write a textbook on the nature of the Tantras.
It should be noted, however, that the true white Tantras teach of the
elimination of all forms of attachments to things by means of properly
psychically cleansing the *nāḍī* system of all forms of gross *prāṇas*
(winds, airs). This cannot be effectively done through the ingestion
of meat toxins. True vegetarianism, coupled with right breathing
techniques (involving *mantras, dhāraṇīs,*[19] etc.), is the method that must
be followed. Nor is it a question of one being attached to vegetarianism,
it is simply a question of not imbibing toxins of any type into the
body and mind. Thereby, pure energies can be evoked and the highest
types of perceptions obtained, such as the 'Clear Light' sustaining
the bliss of an accomplished *yogin.* The *siddhis* derived from meat
intake actually lead to the hell states because they are directly *karma*
invoking, being the effects of the pain caused upon others. The law
subsequently demands that pain (i.e., hell states) must be experienced
before the higher way can be trod.

How can it be otherwise when such callous disregard for the
suffering of sentient beings is presented as a way? If one has manifested
a strong habit pattern regarding something (i.e., an addiction to eating
chocolates, smoking, or promiscuous sex), then one cannot break that
addiction by continuing to perpetually indulge in the act. One must
actually give up the habit, yet our 'Tantric' brothers are making the
absurd claim that by continually eating meat in their practices they can
learn detachment. This is a blatantly hypocritical assertion designed
only to veil one thing; they *are addicted* and have not the capacity to
'give up' their addiction.

The *Fourteen Vajrayāna Precepts* tell us that we are considered to
have broken our *samaya* (or Tantric commitments) if we:

1. Show disrespect for the guru in body, speech, or mind.
2. Have no regard for the rules laid down by the Buddha.

---

19 Meditation aids.

3. Condemn and/or create problems with one's Vajra brothers and sisters.
4. Abandon love for sentient beings.
5. Relinquish *bodhicitta* due to difficulties.
6. Slander the scriptures of Mahāyāna and Vajrayāna.
7. Transmit Tantric teaching without having the proper empowerment and credentials.
8. Abuse and/or foster attachment to the five *skandhas*. (The bundles of aggregates governing the world of appearances.)[20]
9. Harbor skepticism or doubt about the doctrine of Emptiness.
10. Maintain ties to beings with cruel intentions towards Buddha and his teachings.
11. Indulge in accomplishments forgetting the purpose of Vajrayāna practice.
12. Fail to transmit authentic *dharma*.
13. Fail in performance of Tantric ritual practices.
14. Despise or condemn women.

(To these the addendum is generally given, rightly: Upon the foundation of detachment, compassion for other beings is emphasised, especially in the Mahāyāna tradition. Thus, for such a practitioner it is advisable not to eat meat, to avoid inflicting pain on any being and to prevent potential butchers from committing negative actions.

Also, because of the vibration of meat, it can impede an ordinary practitioner from developing great compassion. Therefore, vegetarianism is recommended.)

Now, by observing these fourteen Precepts we see that many are broken through the consumption of meat in one's diet.

The *first precept* works equally well if the guru is on the black or white path, therefore little need further be stated concerning it. If one wishes precise instructions from a teacher, then one must show the proper respect. This is obvious. However, if the 'guru' is giving out false instructions it is right to question the veracity of those instructions without showing disrespect, because the teacher ought to be all wise and knowing with respect to the subject s/he professes to teach. If the teacher is found lacking, then the onus is on the student to seek a

---

20 See my book *The 'Self' or 'Non-Self' in Buddhism* for a detailed explanation of these.

better teacher. Students must never block their enquiring minds. Once the teacher has proved his/her credentials, then students should follow instructions to the best of their abilities. To blindly follow a charlatan (of which there are many, existing both on the physical and psychic realms) is a grievous mistake that may take many lives of painful endeavour to rectify. Therefore, caution should be utilised in choosing such a 'guru'. The fact that such a one is publically accredited does not necessarily prove genuineness, especially in the Highest Yoga Tantras. (For which there really are very few, if any, truly wise and enlightened beings available for the training of the worthy in the world today.)

The *second precept* is directly broken as the Buddha clearly gave us instructions in the *Jīvaka Sutta* (already quoted and commented upon) that meat could *only* be consumed if: 'it has not been seen, heard, or suspected that it was intended for the person'. This precept applied *only for* wandering *bhikkus* travelling from house to house with their begging bowls. It does not in any way apply to modern Tantric practitioners who buy their meat (or have others to buy it for them) from butchers who know full well that the killing is for the monks of that monastery or for the community as a whole within which the monks exist. All yogic practitioners should abide by the spirit of what the Buddha intended and not try to break his intention by contrived arguments so as to be able to fulfil their cravings for meat. This is in effect what the great majority of Buddhists are doing when they use this *sūtra* as an excuse to hold on to their addictions. They use any desired interpretation in order to disguise their craving for meat products.

There are thus Buddhists in Theravādin countries (where meat eating is prevalent), going with their alms bowls to heartily accept meat dishes, without realising that their prime responsibility to their patrons is to rightly educate them to be compassionate. The monastics are not intended to teach lay followers that it is OK to disregard the suffering of sentient beings through accepting from them (without reservation or comment) the effects of products that have caused pain.

A 'non-offending of the benefactors' should not be the prime concern of the monks, but rather they should teach them the proper virtues of following the *buddhadharma* so that they will not have to suffer much further *karma* in later lives. Thus, not to kill should be at the forefront of what they must teach. They are not truly 'detached' when they consume the meat that is endemic in their societies. Rather, they evince attachment to this form of carnal pleasure. Only if they are focussed on right educational practice at all times can they actually be considered to be 'non-attached' (except to the *dharma* itself). This is when they are not at all concerned about themselves, but about others. They should understand that what causes much harm to their benefactors (and inadvertently to themselves) is this propensity to kill. Let them be 100% focussed upon propagating the true white *buddhadharma* (rather than a pallid, contrived version geared to feeding their desires) and therefore not to eschew teaching in confrontational situations. They should rightly use their discriminative mind.

It is an absurdity to think that they do not discriminate when they go about begging for food. Which of them for the sake of 'a non-discriminative mind' would eat a bowl of poison, mud, or acid if it was offered to them whilst begging? Therefore, why do they accept lesser poisons that certainly harm their practices in not so obvious ways? The truth is that they are not honest; they choose to abuse this discretionary allowance of the Buddha's. During the time of the Buddha, society was then overwhelmingly vegetarian, as India remains today. Conversely, modern monastics are practicing in a society that is mostly meat consuming. Therefore, they owe a great obligation to the lives of sentient beings by being a living example of righteousness and foregoing animal meat. They will get nowhere with their practices if they do not rightly discriminate as to the nature of the aggregates they are so willing to burden themselves with.

When Theravādin monks contravene the spirit of the concession made by the Buddha, that is one thing (because the doctrine of *bodhicitta* and the Bodhisattva path is not emphasised). However, for Mahāyānists to repeat the same mistake amounts to a grievous sin because they are supposed to emphasise *bodhicitta* as the backbone of their doctrines. As earlier asked, how can Buddhists assume that it is permissible to eat meat even if 'the animal was not killed by you, or expressly killed for you', and 'that you can freely eat the meat, prefaced by a prayer of gratitude for the life of the animal?' Of course, the animal was killed for you (the consumer), as the butcher had you (the consumer) in mind when slaughtering animals. The butcher may not have had your name in mind, but surely he had your money in his sights – *your money* (or that of your fellow community of monks), for which he will willingly slaughter over and over again. The butcher willingly killed *for you*, because you and your fellow meat eaters have made it worthwhile to do so. A hypocritical 'prayer of gratitude' for the slain being does not expiate your sins. You become steeped in the blood of what you paid to have killed. The *prāṇas* of the death now course in your veins, to inevitably rebound upon you at the earliest karmic opportunity.

The *third precept* is concerned with the workings of a community and is true for those who must establish harmonious relations within such a community.

The *fourth precept* is also broken immediately by the eating of meat, because it means that one abandons such 'love for sentient beings' by being engrossed in direct or indirect acts of harm to such beings. The practitioner may not think s/he has not abandoned such 'love', but the undeniable fact is that s/he *has* through ignorance as to the nature of the effect of his/her actions. A practitioner of the Highest Yoga Tantra should have no consciousness or conscience lapse regarding the way of ignorance, especially in an area so easy to perceive the truth of (if one wishes to and puts forth the effort).

The *fifth precept* is assuredly broken by consuming meat because the practitioner most definitely 'relinquishes *bodhicitta*' due to the difficulties of eschewing the consumption of the products of the slaughterhouse. There is no *bodhicitta* or chance of *bodhicitta* in such disregard of the most basic way that one can cause harm to sentient beings. Millions of concerned vegetarians understand this well, but many of our Buddhist brothers are clueless. They should be their teachers and at the forefront of the education of people as to the way of the generation of *bodhicitta*. They are simply not true Buddhists, if the truth as to what makes a Buddhist is properly analysed. Being compassionate is really the most basic of all the Buddha's precepts.

The *sixth precept* is also broken because they directly 'slander the scriptures of Mahāyāna and Vajrayāna'. This is done by means of presenting definitely unloving teachings, contravening the teachings presented in *shastras* such as the *Śūraṅgama* and *Laṅkavatāra*. Thus they distort the Vajrayāna in such a way that many are led to believe that the causing of great harm to countless sentient beings (especially in the factory style slaughterhouses of today) is correct and right behaviour for Buddhists.

They do not directly or intentionally say this, but that is the effect of their actions and wrong example. It should also be reemphasised that these teachers of *adharma*[21] are responsible for the *karma* of their forms of slander and must suffer the cumulative weight of the suffering they have caused sentient beings because their students are led to believe (in a craftily disguised way) that to continually perpetuate such suffering is justifiable. The law of *karma* is most exacting and *assuredly* manifests in such a way that makes the teacher responsible for the student's *karma* if s/he teaches that which the student is earnestly led to believe. This is especially so when the first precept is emphasised, wherein the student/*bhikksu must* follow the pronouncements of their 'guru'. If the law of *karma* worked differently, then there would be no need for enlightened ones to carefully encode their most esoteric doctrines, for fear of what might happen if unworthy ones developed various types of *siddhis* as a consequence.

The *seventh precept,* the transmitting of Tantric teachings without having the proper empowerment and credentials, is also broken. This is harder to explain, for many present instructors think they have the proper empowerments and credentials, but this is not possible if they in any way eat meat or advocate it, or do not teach the harmfulness of the practice to their students. Put simply, if the teacher does not understand this, he does not really have the proper credentials of being a follower of the Buddha, rather less a guru of the highest of all the esoteric doctrines. This should be obvious by now.[22]

---

21 The proponents of the opposite of what the *dharma*, the spiritual teachings of the Buddha, consists of.

22 In my *Treatise on Mind* series, there are presented many avenues of interpretation to such doctrines and other *kārikās, śāstras,* and *sūtras* that have not yet been conceived of by Buddhist commentators. This will prove that much of what such instructors formerly thought was 'esoteric' is not truly so. (That is, it is 'esoteric' to the way they have exoterically learnt through their lineage, but not in terms of the Universal Dharma that has existed since beginningless time.) I will not dwell on this subject here, as many hundreds of pages of text would need to be presented to prove my statement.

In other words, he may indeed be instructed in the esotericism of a particular tradition, but such teachings are *not truly esoteric* in the light of what is truly 'ear whispered' by genuinely enlightened beings.

The *eighth precept,* the 'abuse and/or fostering attachment to the five *skandhas*, i.e., the world of appearances' *is also broken.* This is because of the refusal to relinquish attachment to the distinctly obvious *saṃskāra* of consuming meat toxins. It should be understood by Buddhists that this type of *saṃskāra* is very difficult to relinquish because it is so deeply seated in the human psyche, having been strongly engendered and continuously reinforced in the most primitive time of human evolution when we were hunter-gatherers. Killing for meat has been a dominant *saṃskāra* fostered for uncountable millennia. The quite sophisticated philosophy and lifestyle of being vegetarian is a much later development, coming in the age when people developed a social conscience.

The bottom line concerning this is that for most people the aggregates that are the hardest to eliminate attachment to are those of the killing of animals and the consumption of their flesh. This, therefore, is what the practitioners of the Highest Yoga Tantra should first demonstrate the mastering of. For this reason, there is the perversion of the Tantras to accept the usage of meat toxins, when the opposite should be the case in order to obey this precept.

Only when the most ancient forms of attachment are eliminated can one think in terms of mastering or conquering the most subtle forms, as Naropa, for instance, had to do when his guru Tilopa asked him to eat the flesh of a corpse.[23] Only when he was in the process of complying did his guru demonstrate that that corpse was an emanation of himself. It was a double aversion for Naropa, both for:

a. being a human corpse, and

b. violating his vow to not eat meat (as all Buddhist monks vowed in those days).

The subtle mastery or relinquishing of attachment of views (erroneous or not) having then been demonstrated, Naropa could

---

23 See *The Life and Teachings of Naropa* by Herbert V Guenther (Shambhala Publications, Inc.) for further detail.

continue with the rest of his testings that would help him gain complete liberation from all of the vicissitudes of *saṃsāra*.

All this said and done, we can say that when one has vowed to never eat the flesh of anything and has done so consistently all of one's life, then such a testing be given by a fully accomplished, liberated master. The *saṃskāras* for each individual are unique and different, as will be evident if one compares the training accorded to Milarepa, Padmasambhava, Naropa, etc. There is however no need for one to do so in this modern era. Now the highly qualified Bodhisattva has many other forms of testings to master that were not really available in Naropa's time.

Where is the Naropa or Tilopa presently incarnate that can be found by enquirers, that can properly teach accomplished Bodhisattvas (or Buddhists for that matter) the higher esoteric truths? True seekers for enlightenment sorely need appropriate testings and teachings upon the path to liberation. (Disciples working upon the lesser *bhūmis* are normally fine with the relatively low level education they get from current spiritual preceptors.) Not understanding the finer points of the teachings of the knotted Tantras, we see present self-styled teachers of the Highest Yoga Tantra present a textbook formula for their students to follow. Why do they act as if they were one of the really great ones incarnate, when this is clearly not so? Let them clean up their own psychic backyard first, to eliminate the greyish *prāṇas* within their *nāḍī* system before they dare to train others in what they have not the proper credentials for.

The *ninth and tenth precepts* need no commenting upon here.

The *eleventh precept* is violated, by indulging in accomplishments that forget the purpose of Vajrayāna practice. How can Buddhists understand the Vajrayāna practice if they do not understand the necessity for the absolute psychic cleanliness of all their subtle and gross bodies *(kośas)?* Their vehicles of experience must become as radiant as the *dharmakāya, sambhoghakāya,* and *nirmāṇakāya* bodies of a Buddha. This is not at all possible if they continuously debase it with foul forms of *prāṇa*. Some of the *prāṇas* may, however, be psychically fouler than meat toxins, such as hatred or vengeance directed against another. Such activities, coupled with *siddhis,* simply makes them masters of the black arts. The *prāṇa* of the slaughter of animals leads in that direction. (As they imbibe the massed fear of the animals being slaughtered, as well as the killing instinct of humans.) They thus enhance a tendency to anger, mental torpor, and the baser types of thoughts.

The 'accomplishments' indulged in make them think that they are masters of the highest of the Tantras, when they have not even mastered the most elementary aspect of the lore of *bodhicitta*, namely to not kill or cause suffering. They are often found revelling in who or what they are purported to have been in a former life, rather than actively demonstrating a higher level of divine activity in this life. (Which should be manifesting, for in reality all lives manifest as a progression to Buddhahood. Thus their accomplishments should be greater in this new life than in an earlier one. This is the only way it can be for an accomplished Bodhisattva, utilising 'skilful means' to rightly educate all those around.) If the teacher has been successful in that form of 'right' education, then all others must also move onwards and upwards to heights supernal. This is the effect of the Bodhisattva vow.

The *twelfth precept* is also violated by meat consuming Buddhists by their failure to transmit authentic *dharma*. How can they transmit the authentic (white) *dharma* when they preach directly or vicariously that the massed breeding and killing of animals for consumption is somehow right? Thereby this also causes great harm to the planet's ecosystem (through methane emissions of cattle, destruction of natural biosystems for factory farming, encroaching desertification, etc.). How can supposed Bodhisattvas be teaching the authentic (white) *dharma* when they teach nothing about relieving animal suffering, nor will they teach the folly to humankind of the effects of the slaughterhouses that have been developed on the earth? It is plainly *adharma* for them to demonstrate and preach so negligently, for which they have much *karma* to reap.

The *thirteenth and fourteenth precepts* speak for themselves and need no comment.

A special quality of the *siddhas* (accomplished perfected ones, Vajrācharyas), is their ability to skilfully use any aspect of the world as a vehicle to liberate themselves and others. This is often referred to as 'skilful means', implying the efficacy of the method used. The Vajrayāna path is the fastest yet hardest way to traverse the way. Very few can maintain the necessary purity and one-pointedness whilst remaining immersed in the material world with all its allurements and distractions from the spiritual path. Such philosophy, like all philosophy, must be applied with special wisdom to withstand the otherwise distortions of the lower self and its desires and justifications for that which it is attached to.

In the Buddhist Tantric tradition, or Vajrayāna, the goal is to transmute one's imperfections and ordinary awareness by means of non-ordinary and also extraordinary methods.

As Geshe Kelsang Gyatso rightfully states:

> Attachment itself, because it is a delusion, cannot be used directly as a path. Even in secret mantra it should ultimately be abandoned. The true practice of secret mantra, in which the bliss arising from attachment meditates on emptiness, overcomes *all* the delusions, including attachment itself.[24]

We must therefore look very honestly at ourselves when justifying the consumption of those things we are attached to. Are we truly using them as a mechanism to meditate on emptiness, or have we merely succumbed to subtler versions of the addictions of the unenlightened man?

It is said that a qualified practitioner of the highest Tantra meditates on the subtle nervous system, and for this, one's bodily elements need to be very strong. Thus, meat is recommended for such a person. Obviously, those that are addicted to meat toxins need meat in their diet because if they try to eliminate it, then forms of sickness will occur, as explained elsewhere. This simply means that first they must learn to become vegetarians (to truly learn nonattachment to such a wrong habit as meat eating) before they even try to become *yogis*. They must learn the lowest of the Tantras first, and when they are ready, they can begin the process of practising the highest of the Tantras. It is ridiculous to feed the body directly with poisons and then to practice 'skilful means' to try to eliminate the poisons. Surely it is best to avoid the toxins in the first place. Indeed, this is what would be expected from one who is on

---

24   Geshe Kelsang Gyatso. *Clear Light of Bliss. Mahamudra in Vajrayana Buddhism* (Wisdom Publications 1982), 9

the road to enlightenment. Is not avoidance of sicknesses and dangers on the path the most skilful way to attain one's goals?

To pretend that one is not attached by consuming meat is a clear case of misconstruing the doctrines of the white *dharma*. It is designed to virtually ensure that the person has no chance of gaining enlightenment. Why should students of Tantra wish to burden themselves with the grossest of energies in order to try to prove that they can overcome it? This is not the course of wisdom in action, and is certainly not the way of *bodhicitta*. It is best always to follow the simplest and quickest way to enlightenment, and this means the elimination of all forms of intoxicants of body (of which the meat consumed certainly is one), speech, and mind. It means the unburdening of all attitudes of mind, and a continuing refinement and transmutation of one's *prāṇas*. Such refinement cannot be achieved by doing the opposite.

One does not pour filth into a clean vessel if one is looking for fresh water to drink, likewise the practitioner of the *authentic* white *dharma* (Tantra) is not *stupid* enough to putrify his/her *nāḍī* system intentionally with foul *prāṇas* and bodily effects. The practitioner is expected to be wise, to be able to utilise skilful means on the path. Neither is one expected to literally fornicate with virginal 15 year old girls, their mothers, sisters, etc., and worse, which many of the Tantras say, if interpreted literally. The proper meaning must first be derived through correct yogic and esoteric interpretation of the texts. Those that advocate such things as the eating of meat certainly do not know what has been encoded into the texts by the enlightened ones of the past. They do not understand the practices of the white *dharma*. Such teachers only know the elements of the black *dharma* that they are espousing, because only the black practitioners (the sorcerers and the like) purposely foul their *nāḍī* systems with their practices.

When practitioners of the Highest Yoga Tantra meditate on their subtle nervous system, they would discover the meat toxins residing therein as a murky substance blocking the flow of enlightening *prāṇas*. The most sensible thing thus to do is immediately eliminate such toxins from their diet. True, they could eliminate it through psychic means, however, there are plenty of other *saṃskāras* to transform as it is. Why make one's task longer and more difficult? After all, the highest Tantric path is also supposed to be the most efficient. The strength of the

Elements in one's body comes from light. It is the quality and intensity of light that one can receive and bear in consciousness that makes one en*light*ened. Vegetable products are formed in light. They capture that sunlight directly, and in this form exist to feed the animal kingdom. The animal kingdom then absorbs that captured sunlight (i.e., *prāṇas)* and converts it into animal *prāṇas* in the dark spaces of their bodies. Such animal *prāṇa* is imbued with the sluggish *(tamasic)* consciousness of the animal form, which is what is ingested when their substance is consumed. Such a sluggish consciousness is the very antithesis of what meditators are endeavouring to produce.

Eating meat has a gradual and negatively engulfing effect on the auric body. The light in the aura comes to be muddied and thickened to such an extent that the direct Clear-Light experience, or its reflection upon the lake of Illumination, cannot be viewed with clarity. Again, why imbue into your system elements that fight, manifest adverse conditionings, to what you are actually trying to produce? Where is the wisdom here? All forms of intoxicants are directly harmful to the unfoldment of the meditation mind and must be strictly avoided.

It is seen, therefore, that the very opposite of 'needing' meat products for the 'body elements' to be made 'very strong' is required for the attainment of enlightenment. (Meaning one's body is full of light – not the darkened *prāṇas* of meat.) Certainly, one's 'body elements' need to be strong, but the practitioner must learn to do this through the complete cleansing from the diet of all toxins and intoxicants as an essential precondition to any form of Tantra. Only when they have obtained strength of body, speech, and mind through 'wholesome foods' should they try to become *siddhas*.

It is irrelevant if this practitioner of Tantra (as it is said) is capable of transforming 'ordinary objects' through meditation on selflessness. Why waste such time and effort, when the goal is enlightenment and the path is supposed to be the most direct? Also, from a (more esoteric) Tantric viewpoint, the *Maṇipūra* (Solar Plexus) *chakra* is the centre of the self-will, wherein the *saṃskāras* of self are generated. This center is directly stimulated by the ingestion of meat toxins, thus if one was truly meditating upon 'selflessness', one would rigorously avoid stimulating this centre, but instead there is the opposite for such practitioners. Again, from the psychic perspective (the nature of the generation of the subtle winds), there is no 'skilful means' evidenced here.

In relation to the excuses for meat consumption, there has also been presented such delusive statements as: 'such a practitioner, by virtue of his/her profound meditation, is not greedily eating meat for his/her own pleasure'. The question always remains, 'if not greedily eating meat', why are they so attached to an obviously non-compassionate act which breaks so many of the precepts of the Vajrayāna?

Though *The Laṅkāvatāra Sūtra* is not of the class of the *Anuttarayoga Tantra* (Highest Yoga Tantra), the Buddha nevertheless gives very clear instructions for such practitioners:

> Mahāmati, when sons or daughters of good family, wishing to exercise themselves in various disciplines such as the attainment of a compassionate heart, the holding a magical formula, or the perfecting of magical knowledge, or starting on a pilgrimage to the Mahāyāna, retire into a cemetery, or to a wilderness, or a forest, where demons gather or frequently approach; or when they attempt to sit on a couch or seat for the exercise; they are hindered [because of their meat eating] from gaining magical powers or from obtaining emancipation. Mahāmati, seeing that thus there are obstacles to the accomplishing of all the practices, let the Bodhisattva, who is desirous of benefitting himself as well as others, wholly refrain from eating meat.[25]

The teaching here is unambiguous and unavoidable for all who would aspire to attain the highest *siddhis* and yogic accomplishment – do not eat meat for any reason. It is antithetical to everything you are aspiring to achieve, unless it is a Rākshasa[26] (a ferocious demon-like entity) you

---

25 From chapter eight of Suzuki's translation of *The Laṅkāvatāra Sūtra*. See also Appendix One.

26 Suzuki's translation of *The Laṅkāvatāra Sūtra* continues with: 'Let not the Yogin eat meat, it is forbidden by myself as well as by the Buddhas; those sentient beings who feed on one another will be reborn among the carnivorous animals. [The meat-eater] is ill-smelling, contemptuous, and born deprived of intelligence...From the womb of Ḍākinī he will be born in the meat eaters' family, and then into the womb of a Rākshasī and a cat; he belongs to the lowest class of men.' Note that a Rākshasa is a demonic being, whilst a Rākshasī is the feminine aspect.

wish to become with respect to the nature of your psychic body, for that is the inevitable effect of the nature of the energies of meat toxins. For then it is the energy of a Rākshasa that you must fight with (because of your wrong habits and attitudes of mind to try to transform). If not transformed it will convert you into a practitioner of the black path.

If such an act causes harm to oneself or any other living beings, more than any good or revelation that may come from it, then what is 'skilful' about employing such means? Neither is the act of drinking alcohol (which is condoned by many Vajrayāna practitioners and teachers). This is nothing more than the insertion of the black *dharma* into the pure white doctrines. It is a grossly twisted and convoluted logic for such activities to be viewed as a means to overcoming one's own concept of 'purity.' Here 'purity' is being seen as something illusional and dualistic, and therefore must be destroyed. Do they mean by this that a Buddha must have the grossest and blackest form of aura in order to be a Buddha, rather than the most intense form of radiance possible? No! Purity of body, speech, and mind are *absolute* musts if one is to try to emulate a Buddha. Only practitioners of the black arts (or the ignorant) denigrate their auras with filthy energy.

As Tantric practitioners we are trying to cleanse all of our *karma* as rapidly as possible. The last thing we want to do is create more *karma,* that according to Buddhist doctrine, will only lead us into hell or other less favourable realms. (Where we will have to start the journey all over again.)

Practitioners advocating meat products should strive to overcome their pride in endeavouring to use 'skilful means' to try to transmute the harm of eating meat. They can substitute simpler practices at the appropriate time. The practitioners of Highest Yoga Tantra should be honest (both to themselves and to others), and say such things as 'it is my pride that prevents me from speaking the truth concerning this subject, that I am addicted to this form of intoxicant. I have not the capacity to overcome this addiction in the now, but I hope that you can learn what not to do by my example. I hope for a better rebirth when I may be able to pursue the pure white Buddha *dharma* and not cause suffering to sentient beings through my actions....'

Other Issues

1) Many claim they get sick when they stop eating meat. A vegetarian diet, however, should not be blamed for this.

It is noted in serious smokers that when they try to stop their addictive habits, sickness often ensues. This is because the lungs are now busily eliminating mucous. This mucous is the result of accumulated toxins that can no longer be sustained in the healthier environment, so it needs to be cleansed from the tissues. The lungs and chest cavity then work in unison to expel what the body no longer needs. Similarly with those who eliminate meat from their diets, the toxins from the coarse substance they have inundated their bodies with come to the surface. These must also be eliminated, producing the sickness that is experienced. Likewise, when one who has lived a careless, dissident lifestyle tries to fast (i.e., drinking only water for a period of time), they also generally suffer sickness as toxins are eliminated from the body. It is a natural expression of what the body must experience when its system is overloaded with deeply ingrained substances that have been stored in fatty tissue and interstitially. These toxins come out all at once, producing the results experienced. Once cleansed, the body is freed from future sickness from such toxins.

Those that experience such detoxification should not, therefore, decry the situation, but rather rejoice in the opportunity to have a far healthier bodily nature. Contrary to the myth instigated by many in the modern medical profession (whose pharmaceutical companies gain enormously from keeping people sick), it is not meat consumption that makes one healthy, but rather a proper balanced diet of fruit, vegetables (including legumes) and nuts. This is the way it is designed to be in Nature. One need only observe an otherwise carnivorous animal instinctually eating vegetable products when they are sick, in order to understand the way things were ordained for all living species.

One cannot simply subtract the meat from one's diet, one needs to replace the missing protein with adequate and abundant vegetable sources. Ask any dedicated vegetarian for recipes and nutritional listings of what constitutes a healthy diet. This information is also very easily sourced on the internet. It should also be noted that in the West, where conspicuous meat eating is prevalent, we witness the tendency of people to go senile as they age. This is due to gross and most base forms of meat and mineral toxins (ingested pharmaceutical chemicals) being stored interstitially, between the cellular structures of the brain, for instance. When they surface at old age in a crystallised form, they damage the brain tissue, retarding proper thought. This is not so with most vegetarians, who generally grow wiser as they age. (Many vegetarians have also had a lifetime of consuming pharmaceutical toxins, and so will suffer the ill effects of these as they age.)

It is best to pay off some of the *karma* immediately for wrong eating habits rather than later, when a more virulent disease will manifest (as a consequence of continued meat eating). First cleanse the toxins, and then begin to understand what it means to maintain good health and a vibrant auric state. Learn the Nature of the lightness (of mind) that comes as a consequence of being freed from meat toxins.

2) 'How could an Eskimo (or any other indigenous human) be a Vegetarian and not lose their cultural identity?'

Such questions are answered simply. We do not ask Eskimos to be vegetarians in the arctic environment they reside in, where the appropriate and respectful culling of animals for the survival of the Eskimo and his family is at stake. Similarly for an indigenous native in the wilderness or natural forest environment they reside in. There is an environmental friendly balance between the hunters and the animals they live with that has existed for untold generations. They are then but a version of a carnivorous animal (such as a lion or tiger) playing an appropriate role in their environment.

We, however, do ask Buddhists to be vegetarians, to be a prime educative example of the right course of action for all of humanity to follow. If an Eskimo became a vegetarian (by becoming Buddhist for example), it would simply involve a change in lifestyle reflecting the more sophisticated thinking process of the philosophy now being embraced. Such a one would however still be an 'Eskimo'. Their lifestyles have already been changed irrevocably since the coming of Europeans into their environment. Many changes have occurred, some not necessarily for the better, however, they are still 'Eskimos'. So also if they became vegetarian, their culture would change somewhat but the fundamental nature of the people would remain the same. 'Why should it be otherwise?' we ask Buddhists and others in our advanced societies.

3) Some argue that killing animals is acceptable because one is only killing aggregates.

Someone possessing such a belief should grab a knife and cut away an arm or leg and see if they are 'only killing aggregates'. Clearly there are more than just 'aggregates' involved in being alive, whether in human or animal form. There is the input of the force of Life itself, plus sentience, or else consciousness, which experiences pain and suffers. Why is there suffering? For humans the answer is relatively simple – to learn to become detached from phenomena (from *saṃsāra* and thereby to gain liberation), as per the Four Noble Truths. But for animals this possibility is *not* open for them. They do not have this thing called 'consciousness'. They simply must learn to live so as to eventually evolve intelligent responses to the impact of the external environment. They learn through pain via simple response mechanisms to avoid certain situations that may occur in their lives.

4) Regarding fanaticism.

This is with regard to whether one should pursue the course of being exceedingly picky as to tiny amounts of meat products in the food one eats. (Referring also to the adulterations and chemicals derived from meat by modern processing methods). The answer is that ideally everyone should tend towards becoming vegan. However, this is not the Noble Middle Way for humanity at this stage. Vegetarianism is, where milk products are permissible. Some milk and milk products, such as cheese, can be consumed in modest amounts, without detriment to health, or creating *karma* of major significance. It is far better, however, to use plant-based milks and tofu as a substitute wherever it is available. This is healthier and is without any karmic ramifications.[27]

---

27   This is also questionable in the light of modern farming methods, the destruction of rainforests to produce many acres of soy crops, and the introduction of genetically modified produce. Truly the captains of our modern agri-business have turned many formerly healthy products into cesspits of future diseases and sicknesses. Organic produce would normally be the answer, but the producers here have generally made

The vegan argument is that in milk products there are many mucous-forming substances that help cause diseases.[28] There is also the consideration of how young animals are treated (calves separated from cows and slaughtered so that the cow can be a milk-producing 'factory'). The argument is valid that there is unnecessary suffering inflicted upon the calves as they must be killed to ensure milk quantities, and that the mother is artificially forced to produce the milk long after she would naturally do so.

Leather products are another case at hand. Leather is an offshoot of the killing industry, thus their use helps contribute to this killing. However, animals are not normally directly killed for their hides (except in the case of the already world-wide discredited fur industry), thus this plays a subsidiary role in the case of animal suffering. Whilst the mass slaughter persists, one can make a case that one can at least honour the animal that was killed through the use of the product in shoes and belts (etc.). For otherwise the skins would be totally wasted, while there is no ill health produced through wearing leather products. (In contradistinction to consuming flesh.) This may seem a facetious argument, especially in the light of alternative products (which normally are not as durable), and this may be so. This is a matter of one's conscience and rational considerations. It is a *secondary* issue to that of the slaughter of animals for meat. Once meat consumption diminishes in our societies, then the usage of the resultant products of their hides also naturally follows suit. Our technocrats may also find better alternatives for this product than much of what presently exist.

The problem also lies in fanatical attitudes. Many vegans can fall into this trap, thereby causing more harm to their psyche, and laying the seeds for sickness, than if they had consumed a little dairy produce. People must realise that energy follows thought. Fanatical or strongly emotional attitudes are generated in the Solar Plexus centre. The forces generated find their outlet in the arenas of the body that the Solar Plexus

---

their produce far more expensive than the commercially available products, making it very difficult for common humanity to afford this produce in an increasing inflationary era. The increasing prices of healthy foods has been one of the success stories of the dark brotherhood (forces of evil) working through the venality of our policy makers and the avaricious in our societies.

28 Cow's milk also has too much calcium, per se, for humans.

centre controls—the stomach, intestines, gall bladder, etc. This lays the groundwork for various ailments to be found in those organs. If the energies are directed upwards to the chest cavity or via the vocal cords (thus projected via the Lung and Throat centres), then inflammatory diseases can manifest there. Cancers of all types can abound in any of these cases, for Cancer is but an abnormally rapid growth of cells caused in part by such strong constant emotionalism. If the fanatical one projects strong thought forms and energies at another, then *karma* is produced that is worse than any *karma* associated with consuming dairy products. Such people must in a future life suffer the reciprocal effects of their energy and thought projections. Beware of undue emotionality, as it is spiritually deadly.

The fanatical (or dogmatic) ones should also realise that they are continuously killing bacteria in their stomachs, or having to deal with and kill various insect pests or slugs in their gardens. This concept was treated earlier regarding previous arguments, such as the fallacy of Buddhists ignoring the 'quality of consciousness' with respect to bugs verses large mammals. It is brought up here to remind the fanatical ones of the unavoidability of killing. There is a natural balance in Nature for all aspects of the living process. Killing or dying is a natural factor in life. There is an entire ecosystem based upon this fact. Humans are on top of the predator list in Nature's kingdoms. This has been so since they invented the weaponry to make it so. The argument thus really is focussed upon the concept of compassion, of what does the least harm to the other, or rather, what is it that best serves the society one is in, and Nature as a whole. The fine balance in this argument of vegetarianism versus veganism really lies in this fact.

One must also consider the existence of dairy farms, or the village cows, where the cows are treated quite conscientiously and humanely. They are left to graze quite contentedly, and know when they are to be milked, to relive the burden of the weight they are carrying. As per usual, the main culprit in the 'pain' factor is modern factory farming upon a mass scale, and the problem of excess male calves. Their culling lies well within the bounds of what a population of such animals would lose if they were in the open savannah with natural predators there. The product from the culling serves the needs of those who are still predatory in their consciousness, and don't think much about the concept of compassion, except within the bounds of their family and friends or human society. They have a long way to go to learn the finer points of the Buddhist concept of *bodhicitta,* and so according to the factor of human free will, which is sacrosanct in the evolutionary process, they have the time to learn. In the meantime, let us educate them the best we can, without fanaticism, but with sane, serene logic, so that over time they too can follow the *dharma* to their enlightenment.

In the meantime, a lot of people earn a living through the dairy industry. They support families and are normally conscientious members of society. Therefore, taking the entire picture into account, there is good *karma* accrued here in the fact of supporting a conscientious and considerately thought out dairy industry. The soymilk ideal, or any similar alternative, would be better, if the entire industry was not taken over by the billionaire class that have introduced genetically modified produce upon us.

Although it may be optimal to be vegan, whether or not one chooses to consume dairy products and eggs is therefore a personal decision. Eggs are karmically a borderline case, as they are not sentient creatures (unless fertilised). Hens lay them constantly, and like cow's milk, they are an animal product that does not harm the animal (although eggs are much more *tamasic).* Nonetheless, in hatcheries the non-egg producing male chicks are often considered an undesired by-product and thus macerated or otherwise killed. Factory farming methods again are the problem of major concern. Free-range eggs, where hens can roam freely, and live normal existences for their species, is what must be espoused. For vegetarians who have an otherwise bad diet (lacking the needed protein, and vitamins), such as most people in India who consume a lot of white rice and greasy foods, then eggs are useful to keep them somewhat healthy.

We can and must strive towards purification to the best of our ability, but without any degree of fanaticism. Otherwise, one will also generate impure *prāṇas* that are destructive to the meditation-Mind and which are consequently sickness-producing.

The ideal of veganism for the majority of people on earth is still far in the future. Therefore, let them first learn vegetarianism. For those with fanatical, finicky minds, it is important that they control their mental-emotional *saṃskāras* rather than going overboard in trying to eliminate every vestige of dairy or meat-derived adulterations from their foods. Stated again, veganism is the ideal and should be aimed for, but not with a fanatical or dogmatic fervour.

Therefore, presently it suffices that one has altered one's attitudes rightly towards being vegetarian and has eliminated all forms of meat products from one's diet. One need not worry about microscopic amounts, any more than worrying about the microorganisms one is continually consuming and killing. In aiming to be Buddhists, one therefore follows the middle way between all extremes. We are not Jains, fanatically trying to stop the inevitability of killing even tiny insects, though certainly we respect all living beings 'as if they were our mothers'. Inevitably, however, this means that a vegetarian aspires to become vegan.

There are three levels of 'extremism' of food consumption that can be viewed here:

1) Extreme meat eating — moderate consumption — vegetarianism
2) Meat consumption — vegetarianism — veganism
3) Veganism — fruitarian — breatharian

Here we see that the vegetarian ideal is the 'middle between extremes'. (Note that fruitarianism[29] and breatharianism are extremes for vegetarians, but will be objects of attainment for certain *yogis* in the future, constituting 'skilful means' for them.)

---

29 Thus there are ova-lacto-vegetarians, lacto-vegetarians, vegans, fruitarians, and supposedly 'breatharians' as the categories of those who try to avoid animal suffering in their diets. In their various ways they aim for optimal health and hopefully a meditative attitude to life. All are viable upon our path. Some might add the occasional 'fish' meal, but such are not vegetarians, but can be near vegetarians. To emphasise, the important thing is to not be fanatical in your eating attitudes. The body easily adjusts to various types of diets. The Noble Middle Way of the Buddha is best in all things. The more one's diet moves towards the fruitarian end of the scale, the greater the energies the individual has to contend with, and unless energy dynamics are properly understood and controlled, then often the energies tend towards producing fanatical and extremisms of various forms, which is also 'unhealthy'.

5) His Holiness the Dalai Lama

His Holiness has encouraged those Tibetans in exile, who now live in countries where vegetables and fruits are more plentiful, to refrain from eating meat whenever possible, although he himself was unable to bear such a diet. He became jaundiced when it was attempted, whereupon his Tibetan physician advised him to discontinue vegetarian practice.

The fact that His Holiness, the great Bodhisattva that he is, understood the need for those in his care to become vegetarians, indicates it is an appropriate teaching for one of his spiritual stature. However, it is unfortunate that his Holiness had such bad advisers when he tried to give up the practice of eating meat, which as a genuinely compassionate being he knew to be wrong. He should have gone to dedicated vegetarians for advice, who knew the art of right nutrition. They could have recommended the best way to overcome the sicknesses that are inevitable when the toxins of meat eating are released (such as by the sudden withdrawal of meat after a life-long habit of meat consumption).

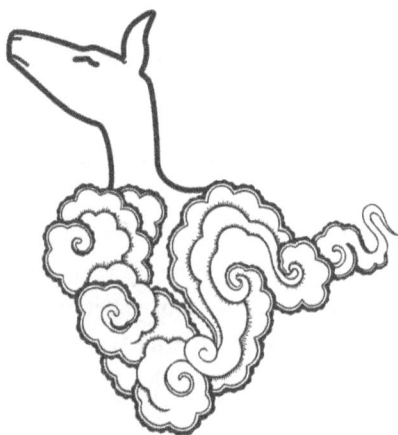

8

An Extract

from the section on Healing from my book
Meditation and the Initiation Process

I have included this modified section from my book on meditation
because the subject of healing and meditation are closely linked to what
feeds an individual. We look to the concept of food as not just physical
food ingested, but also as psychic and emotional-mental forms of stimuli
for the human psyche. They are all *skandhas* and *saṃskāras* that the
individual must utilise in all life activities. I have used the term 'meat
toxins' throughout the last chapter because of the true effect that meat
products have upon a human being, especially concerning the nature
of the maintenance of health.

The detrimental aspects of meat consumption are easily confirmed. For example, heart disease is considered the number one killer in the West. Vegetarians are thirty per cent less likely to die from it, and vegans ninety percent. The second biggest killer is cancer. Vegetarians are forty per cent less likely to develop any form of cancer then their meat eating counterparts, along with a great array of other diseases.[1] Research reveals that meat eaters are more than twice as likely to develop senile dementia than their vegetarian counterparts. Therefore, it is clear that avoiding the consumption of meat is an important step to improving one's health and longevity.

'Health' here does not just refer to bodily health, but also to that form of psychic cleanliness that facilitates the practice of meditation. It is silly to think that the type of food one ingests has no effect upon the health of the body, and consequently upon the ability of one to properly meditate. Though one can learn to meditate whilst being a meat consumer, inevitably the person must learn to transmute the harmful effects of the *prāṇas* ingested via the meat. They are antithetical to the attainment of *bodhicitta,* and to the development of higher, refined states of consciousness. They coarsen, congeal *prāṇas* and debase consciousness and the bodily nature. This is contrary to the refining, rightly energising, and vitalising process of plant substances. Meat products definitely do not facilitate the attainment of enlightenment. Therefore, they should find no place in the life of one who is genuinely aspiring to become enlightened, liberated from all gross sentient states.

The question often asked by the beginner is: 'what has healing got to do with true meditation practices?' The answer will always be the same by the enlightened one – *'everything'.* Right meditation and esoteric healing are virtually synonymous terms, in that one is productive of the other.

The application of the meditative technique must always be healing in its effect, if it is to produce enlightenment-consciousness (the true white *dharma*). The effect is the elimination of everything within the consciousness and threefold personality structure[2] that are associated

---

1   Juliet Gellatley with Tony Wardle, *The Silent Ark*, (Thorsons, 2000).

2   In Buddhistic terms this structure is the body, speech, and mind – the corporeal form, the emotions, and the mental body.

with, or causative of, disease, disharmony, and death. This takes time, much time, for many lifetimes of such conditionings are not easily or quickly eliminated.

The energy that makes enlightenment possible, pouring into the quiescent, awakening personal-I, automatically throws out the grosser substance (of disease) that offers resistance to it. The person must consequently deal with its effects in a conscious way. There are many overlapping cycles of such activity. Progress is made by cleansing the grossest aspects of the physical, emotional, and mental substance, then the subtle aspects, until eventually the being stands transformed, transfigured, and consubstantiated with what is fundamental and integral to being/ non-being. (This is an objective of the entire incarnation process.) Then disease or sickness, as we understand it, is no longer possible.

The detail of this transfiguration process is given as a consequence of practical meditation. The important thing to note is that the key lies in the attitude of impersonality and detachment achieved by the student. The nature of one's mental patterns must change. One must decentralise one's entire thinking process away from the personal 'I' or 'me'. This necessitates embracing concepts of the whole, of one's essential unity with the interrelated multi-dimensional universe, without making oneself the centre of attention therein.

It implies the 'turning about in the deepest seat of consciousness',[3] away from the *lower four* (the centres of consciousness, *chakras* below the diaphragm associated with the field of desire, sensual sensations, and images), to the *higher three* above the diaphragm (the Heart, Throat, and Head centres) wherein the enlightenment-consciousness will be found. The student will later discover that such terms as 'higher three' and 'the lower four' have many levels of interpretation and application. The application of meditation will lead one into many fields of experience, states of awareness, and learning procedures through contact and identification with Beings previously not known.

---

3   See p. 75 of *Foundations of Tibetan Mysticism* by Lama Anagarika Govinda, where he states that: 'It is the reorientation, the new attitude, the turning away from the outside world of objects to the inner world of oneness, of completeness - the all-embracing universality of the mind. It is a new vista, 'a direction of the heart' (as Rilke calls it), an entering into the stream of liberation. It is the only miracle which the Buddha recognized as such and besides which all other *siddhis* are mere play things.'

The 'detachment' that is spoken of here is not what is generally espoused in Vipassana types of meditation teachings, where people are taught to eliminate all types of thoughts from the mind, and to concentrate upon the minutiae of the physical body. This is but a form of forceful denial of impressions coming from sources above and beyond those pertaining to the physical body. A forceful denial or denigration of certain types of thought processes (those deemed not desirable) does not make true detachment. Wisdom comes by means of proper comprehension, through right acceptance and then rejection of what is deemed harmful or not necessary to one's ultimate quest. Once, through wisdom, something is rejected as not necessary, then true detachment is found.

All forms of detachment necessitate discrimination. 'What indeed is right discrimination?' – is what must be asked. In such a case the person may first discriminate what is outside the body from that which is inside. On the inside, we have the discrimination of the organs from their cellular constitution, and then the cellular constitution from the *skandhas*, etc. What is it that makes the 'I' or 'me' is generally the question posed in such techniques. By delving into the minutiae, they cannot find any reality to an 'I' or 'me'. This is all fine, from one perspective. However, no matter how it is dissected in the mind, the human body exists as an integral whole, and must bear the consciousness that does all of the enquiring in this form of meditation. Therefore, the body must be properly fed to support its investigatory activities.

Here 'right discrimination' necessitates the intake of the appropriate foods to facilitate the maintenance of good health, otherwise meditation will not be possible. The concept of detachment then produces an immediate problem to the enquiring mind. The question then becomes: 'should one be detached to the type of food that one intakes into the system?' Often we find this question answered very shallowly indeed. The person generally forgets that right discrimination must always drive all concepts and actions associated with detachment, otherwise the person will not live long enough to gain any form of enlightenment. Thus, what one feeds one's consciousness with, their food intake, is very important. One may say that one does not care about food (through the doctrine of being 'totally detached'), therefore that one will eat either anything, or nothing at all, in order to stay detached. In other words, such a person is choosing not to discriminate between poisons and healthy options, thereby ignoring if harmful disease or sickness producing agents are introduced to the body, or whether the body is nourished enough for him to go on living. Such a course can only lead to disaster for the human individuality. It is not the course of wisdom, and cannot lead to enlightenment, as the Buddha aptly demonstrated when he tried a similar severe form of yogic austerity.

Another example of a form of ignorantly applied detachment is if one decided to be so 'truly' detached as to not care where one is walking at all (that is, to be detached to the nature of the outer environment). So perhaps that one walks lazily across a busy road and gets killed or maimed, or causes others to injure themselves, avoiding him/her. Such a person, by choosing this form of blindness, may simply walk over a cliff and that will be the end for that life.

Clearly, right discrimination is an essential ingredient concerning 'detachment' right from the start. Therefore, not only right food intake, but also what one feeds one's sensory intake with must be properly worked out from the start of one's enquiry as to the nature of 'self'. This includes the thought-forms and emotions concerning one's surroundings, such as what aspects of the multi-media are to be consumed. Dietary wise, the vegetarian ideal therefore logically must become a conscious choice. One cannot simply close one's eyes and ears and remain blind and deaf when practicing the art of detachment. Rather, one must be alert to all incoming sensory data, to learn through right discrimination which to reject and which to accept in one's path to become ultimately wise and liberated from the vicissitudes of *saṃsāra*.

As one learns detachment to those things within *saṃsāra* that inevitably cause pain and suffering to oneself or others, one gets closer to being detached to all forms of illusions *(māyā)*. This is not true detachment until these illusional things are rightly utilised for the purpose of helping all sentient beings gain liberation from suffering, without them becoming props for one's own concept of self-aggrandisement. This is the basis to the skilful means of a Bodhisattva. The realm of *saṃsāra* must become a means or tool to help others gain mastery of phenomena, and of themselves. On this path of Love, one seeks out actions that lead to liberation from *saṃsāra*, not just for oneself but for others as well. In other words, one cannot be detached from the white *dharma*. One must become impersonal in dealings with the all, and yet remain ensconced in Love. How not to be attached to what one must constantly interrelate with becomes an unending meditation for all earnest Bodhisattvas. Inevitably, the meditation is upon how the forces of friction, inertia, strife, and pain in the world as a whole are arrested. The question concerns how one can produce peace and harmony in the midst of strife and conflict. Consequently, the mode of healing all pains within and outside of the bodily consciousness is what concerns the meditator.

Meditation helps one to heal oneself and ultimately the surrounding environment (which is but the extension of one's life in all directions in space). Meditation is the expression of the law of *karma,* which when properly unfolded and taught is based on the paradigm of the laws of evolution. This means that the stages of the unfoldment of meditation will progress in a similar manner to those undertaken by the greater evolutionary space as a whole.

Indeed, evolved Buddhas from long past world-cycles of evolution are in a state of meditation upon their Buddha spheres, which are but spatial universes. Such a meditation-Mind works in, through, and envelopes all that is, and that which must come to be. If the individual on the path to enlightenment is to be freed from the bonds of space-time and the transience of their own personality nature, then they must work to emulate the greater meditation-Mind. Meditation is thus the key to eventual absorption into the spaciousness of the greater Clear Mind of Bliss. For this (and what lies 'beyond') there is no adequate terminology in any language. The comparable Sanskrit terms *śūnyatā* and *moksha* simply translate out as 'the Void'. Later, the *dharmakāya* becomes the focus of awareness.

The attainment of the meditation-Mind, and the resultant internal experiences of one type or another, are concomitant with the number of previous lives spent in pursuit of the Mysteries of being/non-being. For instance, a person may have spent a life in the past learning directly from the Buddha, and later from Jesus, and as the millennia progressed, under a number of other enlightened sages. This acquired experience will greatly assist him/her to quickly master the entire life process and obtain the enlightened Mind in any future life. One tends to quickly catch up where one left off in the past, though within the context of the new cultural and environmental situation.

Such a person would already have been initiated into the associated Mysteries. Nonetheless, former attainments must be recapitulated and then the testings passed in the present life that will allow the surpassing of the high point of the past.

With regard to healing, it will be seen that the true spiritual healer will not ask for money, or any other fee for the healing service. A healer should not profit from another's distress, instead working on a donation basis as an example of giving. Thereby generating the goodwill from patients to meet all future physical plane needs. Ideally, knowledge exists of the karmic interrelationships between the healer and the healed, and that one must work with the laws of Love, colour and sound. At a later stage, to produce the healing a conscious working interrelation manifests with *devas* that embody all manifest Life. The true healer knows that he/she does not really 'heal' as such. Rather, they assist patients to produce their own recovery, and will take pains to teach what mistakes caused the illness in the first place, to try to ensure they are not committed again.

Right education *is always* the true healing practice. This takes much wisdom and skill in action to apply. It should be better understood that the healing of the physical body of its various aches and illnesses is *not the most important thing,* but rather the elimination of the deep-seated karmic causes and related inherited psychological and physiological tendencies from past lives *(saṃskāras).* The healer must begin to truly treat the entire personality and not just the symptoms. The emotional-mental causes of illnesses, specifically of how *the emotions* produce ailments (such as influenza, cancer, and all inflammatory sickness), should be better analysed and treated. A quick fix (whether pills or herbs) is not the true answer, for then similar or worse ailments will crop up later.

Everything must be viewed in terms of *energy,* as all things are constituted thus. This is specifically so with all organisms that are 'alive', and that have their own specific inherent vitality *(jīva)*. There can either be an excessive amount of *jīva* or a dearth thereof. One category of organism (e.g., vitamins) has vitality to give (of varying colourings) and another vampirises (e.g., disease bearing micro-organisms). If the energy to be given is of the type needed by the body, then there is promotion of a vital healthy physical body, whereas if the energy is adverse to the well-being of the body, then there are inflammatory types of diseases (e.g., influenza). If the agent vampirises, such as by some poisons, and bacteria, then diseases of congestion arise (e.g., tuberculosis). This is because as substance builds up so the vital Life is drained away.

Much error has crept into orthodox healing practices through the desire of the healer to keep the body (the form nature) 'alive' at all costs, despite the clear indications of the indwelling consciousness to vacate it. Healers must learn to work with the factor of death as a healing potency, and not against it. This necessitates much meditative insight on the part of the practitioner. Once healers begin to understand and accept the laws of reincarnation and *karma,* they will begin to see the absurdity of many of the quandaries created by such things as euthanasia and treatment of chronically ill, deformed, or totally (mentally) incapacitated patients. There is really no such thing as death, except possibly the 'death' of the human psyche, as a consequence of left hand practices.

The true healer will thus recognise the healing factor in the death of all aspects of the personality, and the teaching value of all illnesses - for *they teach what not to do.* They are caused by the transgressions of the laws of Love and those that govern Life. The patients must be taught to recognise this in themselves. The *karma* always manifests in such a way so as to rightly educate the individual. If the lessons are not learnt, then they will be repeated in another way, until eventually the person learns to do what is right.

It is much like a child learning how to walk, who must fall over many times, sometimes with painful results, before the skill is learnt. The child must also first touch the heat of a flame in order to understand, that although attractive, it is hot and can burn. Millennia-long cycles of karmic unfoldment of sickness, disease, and suffering teach the spiritual child how to walk in the realms of enlightened Being, freed from such ailments. Such a one has fallen into *saṃsāric* involvement and allurement many times, and has learnt to detach from such activity, to pick himself up from the realms of darkness, to enter those of Light. He has been burnt by premature tampering with psychic fires often enough to know what not to do. Consequently, he has become wise and compassionate, recognising the activities in others that cause sicknesses and the like, that have formerly been manifested and now are mastered. He can now rightly offer the cures to those that will listen and are willing also to undergo the disciplines that will produce mastery.

Such enlightened understanding is obviously wellnigh impossible to the materialist and orthodox healers, who will not look at the factor of *karma* and rebirth. These healers will generally manifest contempt and disdain at any suggestion of a subtle energy body, *karma, chakra* system, *devas* or other holistic factors to be taken into account in the healing of diseases.

It should be noted that esoterically we view physical plane incarnation as death, for then the indwelling vital Life 'dies' to the bountiful spiritual realms it is accustomed to. Therefore, death (in conventional terms) is a return to the inner realms, and certainly nothing to be feared.

The arrogance and blinded vision of those trained in Western materialistic ethics and values are a major factor in propagating most aspects of sickness and disease in our societies. This is because true causes are not looked at in totality. Only the symptoms (and secondary disease-bearing factors, as are the microbes and viruses) are examined, upon which the diseases are blamed. When 'causes' are found, then only the most material, concrete ones are considered, such as direct poisons, germs, carcinogenic chemicals, and the like. Other than direct poisons, such things only produce effects *after* the subtle causes have been operating for quite a while, and bodily warnings have gone unheeded. After all, if one produces a cesspool of base energy fields in one's body, then the inevitable effect is the massive breeding of primitive forms of Life that are vitalised by the energy levels of this cesspool. They are the germs (etc.) responsible for disintegration and death, whilst the body has not the vitality to fight off the mass-invader.

People have thus been conditioned to look at the wrong factors as the causes of their distress. Centuries of mass socio-political and materialistic indoctrination have kept them in ignorance, thus laying the fertile ground work for the later concrete factors of disease-bearing organisms that concentrate symptoms at focal points within the body. This forces patients to go to allopathic medical specialists (who are predominantly likewise indoctrinated) who utilise an increasingly sophisticated array of elaborate and costly appliances and technological contrivances to analyse the symptoms, dissect the body, transplant organs, and apply chemicals and the like to effect their 'cures'. For this the patient or health care system must pay the increasingly costly fees demanded.

Surely, true healing must be far simpler, as ordained by the same laws of Life, Light, and Love found throughout Nature. Such healing is engendered by Nature's agents, who originally construed the amazingly ingenious and wondrous human form we reside in. Such laws have been in operation and incorporated in the perfectly integrated universe at large, long before the advent of modern science. Certainly, the many divinely inspired healers knew and utilised them.

Taking a pharmaceutical pill may alleviate the symptoms temporarily, but will do naught to obviate the true causes of disease; it only postpones the inevitable. There are no miracle cures, except those associated with the disciplined self-cleansing activity and purity of lifestyle. In fact, it should be noted that the true healer knows that the healing potency comes not from oneself; one only becomes the *conscious* channel for divine energies *(prāṇas)* after having developed the needed understanding and capacity to do so. The healer adds this energy to the patient who is in the process of healing, and thus effects the cleansing of the diseased areas, or else the healer takes the diseased *prāṇas* into his/her own body, cleansing them with the radiance of the aura he/she possesses. There are also many other healing techniques utilised by true healers. (Limited space prevents us from delving into them here.)

Beware of highly processed factory produced drugs, especially those derived from mineral substances.[4] They are but corpses and skeletons of what was once vital and alive. They produce effects in the

---

4   This is not to say all allopathic medications are bad. Indeed, they are sometimes necessary for acute conditions and certain diseases. However, when possible, holistic healing should always be looked into to work on the deeper conditions behind the disease state, which Western allopathic medicine does not address. Once the subtler conditions have been addressed (i.e., repressed emotionality), outward manifestations of disease can resolve themselves.

now, but postpone the inevitable. The *karma* of the postponed sickness will simply come out in another more virulent form in another part of the body at a later time, or in a later life. The true healers, here, are the greater *devas* (solar *devas*)[5] working via the doctors, and they use these 'corpses' as the foci for their work. The *devas* are the angels of Christianity, or the *ḍākinīs* and *ghandharvas* (etc.) of Buddhism. These *devas* are omnipresent, and can be contacted consciously via right meditation techniques.

The psychic emanations from 'corpses' are effective in producing their own types of symptoms of disease, and in time *must* be eliminated from the living vital tissue. When done so, they will tend to produce further sicknesses. The patient goes to doctors for further chemotherapy, artificial hearts and the like, and so the cycle continues. True meditation techniques will give one conscious contact with the angelic forces, as healing *devas* are always predisposed to work with those that care for the formed realms (which they embody). Their work is greatly facilitated by conscious co-operators. Such co-operative endeavour is the way of the medical profession of the future.

The main points to consider in meditative healing are thus:

- Beware of the critical mind, irritability, fears, and all forms of emotional extremism, as they are major factors in devitalising the body (as energy is expended and dissipated in the emotional and vital bodies) and thus the production of illnesses.

---

5   See Lama Anagarika Govinda's *Foundations of Tibetan Mysticism*, p. 111 where he states that 'the Tibetan word *'lha'*, which generally corresponds to the Indian word *'deva'*, i.e., an inhabitant of higher planes of existence (comparable to the Christian Hierarchies of angels) is used also for *Dhyāni-Buddhas* and *-Bodhisattvas'*. The lesser *devas* are the fairies, pixies, nature spirits (etc.), however, the greater *devas* specifically concerned with this healing work are self-conscious, of equal or greater 'intelligence' than humans, and could be better equated with the *ḍākinīs* of Tibetan Buddhism. Govinda explains (on p. 190) that *ḍākinīs* are 'female embodiments of knowledge and magic power who - either in human or super-human form - played an important role in the lives of the *Siddhas'*. Further (on p. 192) he states that 'thus *ḍākinīs* become the genii of meditation, spiritual helpers, who inspired the *sadahaka* and roused him from the illusion of worldly contentment. They were forces that awakened the dormant qualities of mind and soul.'

- Beware of the ingestion of chemicalised, devitalised, and highly processed foods, all forms of drugs, psychoactive substances, narcotics and stimulants. These either devitalise or poison the body, causing areas therein for the breeding of disease bearing factors.

- Beware of the ingestion of animal products, too much fat, sugar, carbohydrates, and all forms of fast foods, fad foods, and high-priced gimmicks (vitamins, etc.) with which many overload their digestive and eliminative systems. What the body can't properly digest (or must utilise much energy to convert and store, such as in fatty tissue) acts to devitalise it. The animal products also debase the body with low-grade *prāṇas* that are antithetical to the production of refined, higher states of awareness.

- Eat simply and wisely the products that have ripened in the sun, and enjoy what you eat.

- Listen well to the body, it will tell you when sicknesses are approaching. Learn to fast, abstaining from all solid foods and especially to bouts of emotionality when sickness approaches. Then you will learn to quickly heal yourself with a minimum of cost and maximum effectiveness. The fasting allows the body to direct the sum of its vital forces to rectify the imbalances and disease in the areas of need. That is what the healing factors in the body have been designed to do.

- Work with the body's natural defences as much as possible, developing peace of mind and a meditative lifestyle, knowing well that most sicknesses are but the effects of wrong actions in thought, word, or deed. They will pass once the true causes have been ascertained and eliminated. Look specifically to the emotional body, for most diseases (especially cancers, inflammations, and fevers) stem from constant emotional activity. This concerns the continuous agitation of auric substance (centred upon the Solar Plexus centre), the endocrine glands, and the areas of influence in the body that they control.

- Specialised attention may, however, be needed in cases where long periods of bad eating habits, toxin intake, and 'riotous' lifestyle, have caused major abnormalities to manifest in the bodily organism.[6]

- Live as much as possible in harmony with all of the laws of Life, which naturally govern all biological processes. The central factor of which is the sun, with its Life-giving waves of light. Light is the factor underlying all that we can come to know. Plants exist specifically to capture sunlight and convert it to the starch, proteins, etc., that animals need to sustain their lives. This is part of the reason for the need of a vegetarian regimen in one's lifestyle if one wishes to avoid diseases, as plants offer a direct source of sun-like vitality needed for good health, whilst animals offer a debased secondary source, adulterated with its own oft diseased emanatory *prāṇas,* fears and associated toxins.

- The law of *karma* is but an emanation of the rectifying influence of the greater Sun at the Heart of all Life, ruling over all of the imbalances of the energy equation in the environment, of the bodily nature of the universe as a whole. To be able to heal oneself, in Truth, one must therefore learn (via a meditative lifestyle) to:

    a. Be *serene* enough to listen to the silent voice of the conscience (which is but a touch of revelation from this Heart of Life) when it manifests, so as to be able to rightly avoid bad decisions that would be productive of *karma* that would have to be cleansed later.

    b. Be *alert* to the possibilities of the manifestation of the rectifying waves of *karma,* and thus offer no hindering action to their outcome (seemingly either good or bad as far as our personality desires are concerned).

    c. Be sensitively *alive* to the impacts of streams of vital health-giving light and revelations from higher sources that are healing in their effect.

    d. Thereby to *watch* carefully the effects of all one's actions in the material world that would sow the seeds of disease or disharmony (to sprout sickly weeds in the future).

---

6   Many books by members of the alternate medical profession are also helpful, especially those espousing a vegetarian lifestyle.

To be serene, alert, alive, and to constantly watch the effects of one's actions in the ephemeral world are some of the major outcomes of the practice of meditation, and we can clearly see that a healthy mind really concerns the production of emanatory good health far and wide – expanding to the sum total of all that the mind contacts and influences. This is more than just the physical body of the being concerned, it refers to every modulation in the fabric of Life whereupon the energies and karmic streams associated with that mind must affect and effect. These streams come from the past and are modulated in the ever-present bath of energy impacts that is the eternal Now, and which the organising consciousness (that is the meditating mind) projects in such a way that future events mould a pathway that the embodied form must follow.

This embodied form is our personality structure, and if one follows without hindrance or resistance the pathway of the projected energy modulations, then perfect health is ensured. Such a being is deemed enlightened, a divine healer. However, if there is resistance to these modulations then we have friction, heat, and consequent pain. This grinding inertia is productive of disease. Lack of conscious understanding (of the way of manifesting ephemerality all around) is the normal way of those bound to the personality world. Such beings are moulded by the past and resist that which the future ordains for them. Thus is ignorance fostered, and from ignorance comes the host of diseases, the world of suffering that people know well.

What I have described here is really the background to the Buddhist concept of the twelvefold formula of Dependent Origination, which is claimed to be the basis of the perpetual cycle of births and deaths, and has its basis in ignorance *(avidya),* a non-recognition of reality, which is responsible for our present state of consciousness. The Buddha asked, as *Govinda* points out, the simple question:

> 'What is it that makes old age and death possible?' And the answer was: 'On account of being born, we suffer old-age and death!' Similarly, birth is dependent on the process of becoming, and this process would not have been set in motion, if there had not been a will to live and a clinging to the corresponding forms of life. This clinging is due to craving, due to unquenchable 'thirst' after the objects of sense-enjoyment, and this again is conditioned by feeling (by discerning

agreeable and disagreeable sensations). Feeling, on the other hand, is only possible by the contact of the senses with their corresponding objects. The senses are based on a psycho-physical organism, and the latter can only arise if there is consciousness! Consciousness, however, in the individually limited form of ours, is conditioned by individual, egocentric activity (during countless previous forms of existence), and such activity is only possible as long as we are caught in the illusion of our separate egohood.[7]

The production of 'perfect health' is therefore the way that one can escape this wheel of Dependent Origination. It is a means whereby that which is not the 'self' can be identified and merged with. Eliminating egocentric activity eliminates the causes for disease, and the need for rebirth into cycles of suffering.

When seeking for those who purport to heal human woes, look always to the true motives of the healer concerned: what the healer gains personally, and what is done unselfishly for the good of others. True humbleness and right motive, zealously applied on the path of Love, guarantees success. For humbleness leads one eventually to the highest teachings, and right motives to truthful Revelations. Success, however, is not necessarily what the aspiring one imagined it might be at the beginning of his/her journeying.

7   *Foundations of Tibetan Mysticism*, 245.

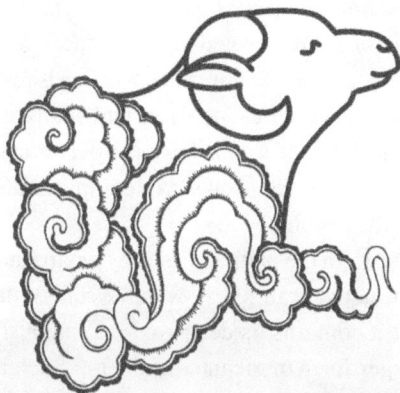

9

Environmental Considerations

Humanity's desire for meat causes great suffering on plants, animals, and humans. The eating of meat is not only responsible for the mass unnecessary slaughter of all these innocents, but also of the deforestation of countries for farmland (e.g., the Brazilian rainforests). The earth was once fully forested, but the forests have been largely destroyed by felling and burning. The *karma* for this still remains potent today. The deforested land has often degraded further, sometimes towards producing deserts, because of general overgrazing. Deforestation has increased exponentially over recent decades. A point that should be made is that if a forest was cleared even as long as 80 years ago, the land it grew upon oft remains degraded today. It takes considerable time for a forest to regenerate to pristine or near pristine conditions.

Humanity's *karma* even engenders the mass starving of millions of people throughout poor countries who do not get enough food to eat, and much of this is attributable to cattle and sheep farming. The same land could more sanely be utilised to feed vaster quantities of people through vegetable foods. One acre of land devoted to the growing of protein through walnuts, for instance, will feed approximately 20 times more people than one acre devoted to beef cattle.[1]

Often in poor countries the government officials resume a policy of selling their exports to America, or places with high capital investment stratagems. Meanwhile, the grains from the poorer countries are sent to feed the cattle during the snowy winters in the USA, rather than directly feeding the people.

There is a truism in the platitude used by environmental groups in the West that one acre of rainforest, with the sum of the wild-life and eco-system that it contains, is destroyed continuously to make one meagre hamburger for American consumers.[2] Such action actually starves millions each year, preventing proper nutrition and the skilful utilisation of the world's resources, as people in Third World countries often live on a subsistence level and can barely produce enough food for

---

1   'As nutritionists such as Dr Frey Ellis and Prof J. W. T. Dickerson have made abundantly clear, plant foods are not only absurdly undervalued for their nutritional worth, but if fed directly to man rather than after processing through animals they can increase the nutritive yield per acre by up to ten fold. Soya beans, for example, yield seven times as much amino acid per acre as milk production and eight times as much as egg production. An animal must consume seven plant calories in order to produce one calorie's worth of human food....An acre of walnuts will supply more than 1000 pounds of shelled meats with a food value of 3,000,000 calories. This is twenty times the amount the same acre would yield in beef. The protein quality of the nuts would be as great as in beef and of superior quality. It is to man's shame that these values in nuts and pulses have been ignored for so long by those whose eating pattern has been under the thumb of the powerful meat industry and Western man's preference for eating flesh.' Jon Wynne-Tyson, *Food for a Future*, (Abacus, 1976), 84-9.

2   150 acres of tropical rainforests are destroyed each day; 1/3 of which are cleared for large-scale cattle ranching. For every burger produced from the Central American rainforest, 55 square feet of forest is devastated. (*Sierra*, March 1995, page 26.)

Around 260 million acres of forest in the United States alone have been cleared to produce a meat-centred diet. It is estimated that every person who adopts a pure vegetarian diet saves one acre of trees per year. (Fall 1996, *Mothering,* page. 64.) See Appendix III for further detail.

themselves in order to host the multinational meat industry. Cattle and sheep are big money earners for these countries, often used to pay off their massive national debts to such organisations as the World Bank. If this lower subsistence level could be properly understood in terms of protein that any country is lacking (in relation to the whole world's supply of it), then the malnutrition caused by the rich West buying the grain of the poorest countries to feed cows during winters would be resoundingly condemned and cease to be. In effect, America (or similar rich countries) are the bully countries of this (and last) century, as a related consequence of aggressive meat consumption and related *karma*. If many have to starve because you eat your cow, wouldn't you want to change for a better diet if you were at all compassionate?

Centuries of wastage of food have gone by so far. Daughters and sons starve because the masses of people are led to consume meat, the least productive of all types of food in terms of yield per acre. Overgrazing all over the world produces a rapidly creeping forward of planetary desertification. Meat eating as a sensory act is retrogressive for the true human spirit and its advancement to higher consciousness states. Such eating habits are undignified in their mannerism, throwing us back to the primitive social status of hunter-gatherers, rather than of being sophisticated, civilised beings worthy of a high civilisation with morally sound ethics. Meat consumption is a drain on a society's general health, bad for the environment, and non-preserving of Nature.

The defenceless animal kingdom are tormented, maimed, and buried in this cruel form of capital punishment. Based on past beliefs and methods preserved by humanity, all three kingdoms (plants, animals, and humans) suffer. We are energetically surrounding ourselves with death (and corpses have never been deemed hygienic).

The effect of these industries on the world is horrific, with mass propaganda aimed at people doubling and tripling their annual intake of meat, and encouraging wastage, force-feeding of animals, hormone injections, and the overcrowding seen in modern intensive animal-farming methods; all for current product market value, and money making strategies.

There are many in the Buddhist society who ignorantly do not realise the harmful nature world wide of the meat industry. Thereby they subserviently aid the quest for profiteering by rich corporations, thriving upon the bloody carcasses of myriads of animals. Elsewhere in the world, the poor are undernourished and starve for lack of basic food needs, when a superabundance of food could be produced for all, on land that is inadequately utilised by the greedy impetus of the modern cattle and sheep farming industries.[3]

The greed that is demonstrated by this model is ethically unconscionable and environmentally unsustainable. A system should thus be constructed to work out the appalling cost ineffectiveness of eating meat as a food source for countries. Aside from cattle farms, the battery chicken factory is a grotesque fashion in the meat industry. Thankfully, descriptions of the gruesome fate of these wretched inmates now deter some humans from the misuse and mistreatment of animals. Perhaps organisations for the prevention of the cruelty of animals should work more potently to produce real changes here? The systems used currently for the indoctrination of social culture to normalise slaughterhouses is barbaric and should be outdated in this modern civilisation.

---

3   'Think for a moment what the habit of meat-eating involves in terms of the world's food supplies. It means the extensive growing of crops, notably grain, in order to feed animals, which after an expensive interval we take back in absurdly disproportionate quality and quantity of food in a form that we hallow, quite incorrectly, as being far superior to the plant-life from which it was derived. In addition to being fed the corn that requires great tracts of the world's land supply, the animals themselves, even in these days of 'factory farming', still need further huge areas for pasture.

About four-fifths of the world's agricultural land is used for feeding animals, and only about one-fifth for feeding man directly.....It should be added that this grossly inequitable situation is being worsened by the advent of factory-farming which is producing a population explosion of animals as providers of human food that is outstripping the human population explosion as a galloping competition for the basic plant foods.

When we consider the work and cost and wastage that goes into stock-breeding in order that the world's affluent minority can indulge so unnecessary a luxury, the sheer extravagance and foolishness of it all is staggering. We read in our newspapers about the starving and under-fed millions, and all the time we are feeding to meat-producing animals the very crops that could more than eradicate the world food shortage; also, we are importing from starving nations large quantities of grain and other foods that are then fed to our animals instead of to the populations who produce them.' Jon Wynne-Tyson, *Food for a Future*, The Ecological Priority of a Humane Diet, (Abacus, 1976), 16-17.

As previously mentioned, the consequent freeing of land could be increasingly used for more crops of local green produce to feed more people better food. It is saddening to think of the effects of the modern era's farming being wastefully mismanaged for mass commercial carcass production.

The current system, which increases the residual toxins in the body, such as rampant herbicide, pesticide, and fungicide use in crops (which become bioaccumulated in animals who feed on it) is far outdated by saner methods of natural farming (of biodynamics, organic farming and permaculture). Is it not so hard to see that the environment we are living in affects us? Are we so childish to think that the environment is too huge to be affected by our actions upon it?

Are we trapped in a fundamentally small paradigm of thinking, the way people thought (such as when the world was presumed to be flat and at the centre of the known universe) before pioneers like Galileo and Christopher Columbus brought their revelations? The extension of this thinking is that the planet is a large place, far larger than our individual actions. We are dwarfed by our planet in size, but our actions as a collective whole have a cumulative effect. This is an extremely simple mathematical equation.

Are we so awe-struck by scientific inventions and technological discoveries (such as space travel, perhaps as a reaction to once thinking of ourselves as being at the centre of the universe) that we have now lost all responsibility in our thinking concerning the integrated bio-diversity of this planet? Do we feel surrounded by such vast space, and feel such a small part of this universe, perhaps even insignificantly so, that what we do to our fellow creatures matters so little to us?

What type of psychological flaws might we find here in humanity, being blinded to the destructive role that meat eating has upon the environment in which we live? People must turn around their thinking here, just as they had to do when they discovered that the earth is not the centre of the universe. Although earth is now accepted as not being worthy to have the sun revolving around it, humanity still acts as if they are at the centre of our universe (free to take what it wants). An effect of pridefully being at the centre is the disregard of environmental factors and of other species. Is it only when the environment threatens one's life that one suddenly finds a purpose to live in harmony with the surrounding sentient life forms. People can then learn to either:

1. Explain logically that humanity as a species is not the centrally evolved life form. If this is found to be the case, then humans should start to care for the environment better so that they do not internally poison the earth (and themselves along with it).

2. Think of themselves as at the centre after all, and if this is the case, they should have stopped their negative actions upon the rest of the environment, and started working like the metaphor of a 'good king'.

Humanity's current collective psychology towards animals can thus be paralleled with the ontology of an unjust, badly ruling child king. The unthinkable effects from his purposefully avaricious actions and greed include raping the planet for meat toxins and for material comforts. The planet is thus in dreadful shape and the only escape plan seems to be to travel in a spaceship or time capsule, irresponsibly leaving this mess to be fixed up one day in the future. The child king wants to live on, with this planet ruined. Will he grow up to listen to a responsible voice and become more inherently lovingly active, aware, and wisely astute as to the consequences of his actions?

What is meant here, is if he decided to be a bad king (by having dominion and priority over all other species), due to his psychological make-up, he thus may act to orchestrate butchering (to be the good king's opponent). Despite irresponsibly acting (as many rulers of the past and present do, through the psychology of being the central all-powerful figure), then the resultant cumulative detrimental effects would be deemed okay in his thinking (assuming such effects don't ultimately affect him personally). This however will not be the case, in reality, for the inevitable effect is increasing senility, or the increase of detrimental bodily toxins that inevitably cause debilitating sickness, plus later karmic consequences.

The earth's fate is indelibly linked to humanity, and inextricably entwined are their histories, but humanity is a 'king' that has custodianship of the earth. Their rulership is currently to the detriment of all life forms on the planet, through needless consumption and destruction of the streams of life thereon.

Esoterically, the physical plane is not at the centre of the spectrum of Life in the universe. Will humanity also recognise this? How will they react (once they discover this paradigm) to new subjective discoveries of science, to the harm that the meat industry causes to the planet's ecosystem, or to recognising the existence of Lives other than those apparent to the physical senses? This will be possible once consciousness is clarified with the vital purifying *prāṇas* from the plant kingdom alone, allied with the right concentration on compassionate thought needed to bring in intense light from sources beyond the physical sun.

If human history was understood to be indelibly linked to the earth's history as part of a multidimensional universe, then there would be the manufacturing of a proper interpretation of history and a better understanding of the earth's future (of where we are all going). Historians and prophesiers (future gazers) will have to reinterpret much after learning so many new subjective (cosmic) facts once they have become enlightened. They will learn that all is governed and interrelated by the energy of Love, and that the path of compassion is the only way out from the suffering found upon this planet. They will learn that their fate and that of the planet is directly linked. They will learn that the nature of their new understanding of the process of active compassion is a journeying on the gift wave of Love, to be absorbed in a unified, multidimensional universe of meaning. They will learn of liberation from form and formed concepts – taking a journey to That which is beyond (consciousness itself). They will learn that this is the only true way to travel into the depths of space. They will learn that such travel is Void of self, of the kingly pursuits and all related images that must be left far behind them.

Before proceeding further, let us briefly turn our gaze to the bold and self-centred atheist psychology of Westerners (an imposed materialistic-nihilistic religion of the masses). It is learning with no purpose, no significance, no reason. It describes us as hopelessly small in a vast universe, emphasising the idea that we might be alone in the universe to make us special (and therefore with only ourselves to keep us happy). As if being the only race of our kind in this daunting space adds some value back to this miserable and often speculative human psychology. 'If there is only us to account for in the equation of all that is', they think, 'then why not kill other sentient creatures for our own consumption? What does their pain matter anyway if they can be sacrificed for our carnal desires?' Is there any real difference in the effect here between the atheist's mind and actions and that of the meat-eating Buddhists? Surely our thinking has rebelled, going from the other extreme of the earth being the centre of the universe, into a nonchalant attitude, oblivious of the effects of our actions due to our relatively perceived smallness.

What is perceived is one's own inherently selfish thinking and a self-image stemming from the psychological indoctrination of living in predominantly non-loving, materialistic, atheistic countries. The majority of the world's rapidly rising population, numbering now (as of 2023) approximately eight billion, are often bombarded with significant lying propaganda extolling the 'virtues' of meat consumption. People are distracted from basic ethical questions because of their fascination and worship of the technological wonders of this materialistic age. Thus they take on board the unwholesome atheistic-nihilistic practice of animal sacrifice for human greed as an adjunct to their God of material consumption.

Is Nature balanced? Is there an intelligent life form of order reigning over the ecosystems of the planet? Is it co-operational? Does it work according to law with the physical constitution of a human and humanity? These are important questions. If we could give our minds a rest, and start to laugh a little, we might notice the inherent selfishness of this small human race sitting on the earth, with its disappointingly self centred compulsion for daily pursuits of physical pleasure. In a culture where food is so readily accessible, better trains of thought should also be available for people to develop the wisdom to deduce healthy dietary considerations, based upon truthful information, taking the environment into full consideration. They should inevitably learn to live without excessive desire for material possessions, and begin to think on more subtle levels, as to the where's and why's of food produce and excessive animal slaughtering, and its true effect on our modern society.

Who knows, perhaps the laws of compassion could be cleverly fixed in the consciousness through the right will of the people. If we all were to eat just grains, nuts, fruit and vegetables, we would live twice as long in terms of our ability to clearly think. Likewise, the cow (or sheep, or goat, etc.) that now suffers the butcher's knife would live also.

There is no necessity for subsistence living. (Particularly in the countries that eat meat.) The wealthy countries generally consume more meat, yet they have the least excuse, as they are much better educated than their brothers/sisters in poorer countries. They need to see that little is of worth in our society when pain is continually projected onto lambs (and cattle, etc.). Little value is knowledge when the process of our development requires killing. Little is of worth when the shelves are packed with processed meat products and we see refrigerated bits of abattoir victims. The exhibition of human compassion in society amounts to very little, and particularly those eating meat can or should be blamed. Those who eat meat are a menace to the natural animal life of their countries, or any other we wish to view. Natural living requires unaffected living, and cattle farms, etc., are certainly not unaffected, because compassion as a quality is not existent there. These numerous cattle are designed to be eaten and to feed all those consumers with fork and knife (ready to gnaw). A sexual perversity is this desire for meat, this desire to be at one with the animal kingdom in this way. Little is known by average humanity about its effects upon childhood, of the great effects of *karma* produced, in thus feeding the world's children and keeping their homes unmeritorious in form.

The butcheries continue to manufacture their meat products regardless. They continue to carve the specimens of meat into neatly presented squared, cornered packages. People drive around in cars, spoiling the planet, as they continue to dine out in a restaurant upon all available meats with their regular fouling habits; chewing upon legs and dead chickens, swallowing meat offal in burgers, hooves put through the grinder, the oceans ravaged for fish, etc. The process continues, of the rampant disregard for the plight of animals and their sufferings.

There is a notion that pigs are better when they are properly shaved, rid of hair, and baked and boiled in a vat of fat and pulled out, jellied and flat. Very few regularly stop to think to check the true price of this unassuming monstrosity, of the 5.65 Kg ham. Where do the piglets end, perpetually born and fattened for the next chew in a human mouth? How do humans expect to cleanse *karma* when they are perpetually making it? These murder victims exist upon a far greater scale than what the ignorant consumer ever actually conceives. A truly endemic holocaust of suffering continuously exists right before everyone's eyes, but very few care enough to do much about it. The crimes keep on recurring, and try as we might, people still buy cars and drive them to the shop where they buy their ham and other parts of animal remains. This charade of 'civilisation' continues while humans pretend to care about the environment and the planet as a whole, but conveniently ignore the suffering they cause every time they chew upon a carcass.

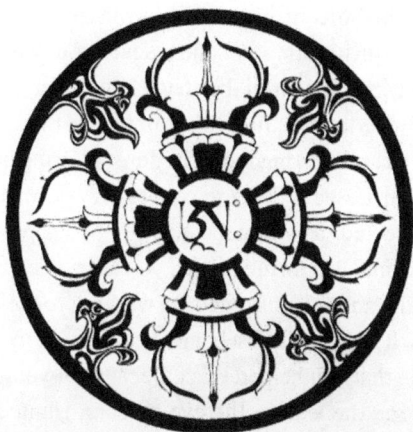

10

Conclusion

Put your picket signs up if you are a truly compassionate Buddhist trying to walk the Bodhisattva path; do your part to help end the war against animals. Of course, this war is a little one sided, but many forget that it is actually a war and that the animals are the innocent casualties. There is no Geneva convention to best look after these prisoners of human predatoriness, so people continue to entertain and feed themselves on the slaughtered bodies of those whom they have captured and then bred for their gluttony.

We wonder how many children would actually like meat eating if it was obligatory for them to take a trip to the abattoirs and see their favourite pets being slaughtered for human consumption? They have more sense than their parents who force them to eat such unsavoury produce, supposedly for their 'health'. But people do not have the compassion to truly inspect and inquire as to why this massed butchery continues. They simply obey the indoctrination of the vested interests that make their billions of dollars from massed animal suffering. Therefore, people turn a blind eye and a deaf ear to what they will not see and hear, staying content in the status quo of complacency.

Humanity, woe to you that you don't hear the screams of the agonised, tortured animal kingdom. They are suffering because of your blindness and heartlessness. They scream as they become your aperitif, so 'tastefully selected' as you delicately grill your prized carcass to disguise your shame. It is fortunate that you are not actually splattered in the blood of the animal consumed, or walking in the urine that you caused it to spill. It breathes its last breath before being messily beheaded on the guillotine that you helped erect, because of your lust for flesh.

You do not see the lean in the eye (vacant, slanted thinking) of the grandmother who chops and stores meat portions for a living, or feel the pain in her muscles and bones. You would also not clean the floors of an abattoir, and like in a barbershop pick up the last locks of an animal's hair. Sweep, sweep it all into a bundle of joy. Have your dinner deposited in front of you, somehow trying to remind you of your ill will and lack of compassion for your fellow beings. So, what is it that can teach you compassion? Do not pretend to be a peace activist or compassionate person whilst you harbour such ill will against innocent beings. Every act of the guillotine of conscious thinking comes crashing down to measure your 'humanity'.

Do not pretend to be a soul afraid of *karma,* or fear the visit to the doctor's office, when your every action in the consumption of slaughtered beasts brings you closer to requital. The fingers of *karma* are already starting to work in your lungs and your bodily organs. If you look carefully, you will find this to be the effect of your meat eating, of the blood *karma* of killing too many beings. Your increasing senility may prevent you from consciously registering this fact, because you will deny what can be clearly seen clairvoyantly (and worked out so logically). You will deny because you care not about your part in the continued slaughter, and you are addicted to the acquired taste for the product of your desires. Nevertheless, *karma* continues to work its hand upon you – it does not stop. When you do get sick, you need only look to your acquired taste for the cause of your pain.

On your summer holiday, look deep into the pool and catch the gaze of the soulful eye of a fish. Net it and do not throw it back. Let it wriggle in the air as you enjoy this animal's death, it's vital energy is what you will live on. To put it bluntly, your killing habit fills your lungs with death, supporting your next mercenary effect upon the animal kingdom. So you encounter death again and again, and the continuation of the *karma* of all that you have needlessly killed. If only you had been a little more observant prior to this warning. Be now warned. Death is the message ascertained by your willingness to kill all creatures, large and small (if they taste good in the mouth). Harness the energy of death in your appointment with *karma,* and see who eventually wins, the lamb or you? Do you care? You will when you suffer the *karma* for the pain of all the animals that you have passed carelessly through your mouth. Chew these words thoughtfully. When eating, am I preserving a holistic decision to preserve Life, or am I making a mockery of my own? What do I receive (recurringly) when I constantly amputate an animal's ability to utilise their legs with no reason but to preserve mine for walking. Where will I walk when there is no more meat left to eat? To the garden patch, I will go, I will survive. I'll eat vegetables, and there starts my fresh day of living.

If we look at the psychology of meat eating, we find it not much different to that of the one who plots a murder, where the essential determinant in their act is to order a hired killer (a 'hit man' or butcher). A Buddhist who ignorantly thinks that this causes no *karma,* due to repetitively praying (intoning *mantras)* for the deceased animal's soul, is ludicrously and preposterously lying to his or herself. If the rest of humanity thought in terms of such a method of expiation, then a killer could be exonerated if s/he spoke kindly of the victim, or by giving prayers for the victim's Soul. The consumer has little or no concern when it comes to killing animals, as one does not see much need for accountability in the grocery store. There are no signs indicating the amount of *karma* to be paid back.

Noticing the psychological aspects here, once again it should be pointed out that *karma* is formed by the intention to eat meat. The *karma* of eating meat produces the intention to kill animals and thus the hiring of a killer. This killer is defined by the desire to eat meat (the desire itself being the killer), and the *karma* is metered out according to the strength of the desire. If the Buddhists as a collective whole changed by properly observing the nature of truly compassionate thinking, then each day thousands of animals would be saved from their fate of being chopped under the knife. The place of dwelling then of these animals (e.g., their graves) would no longer become the belly of the consumer - or the Buddhist's belly. That belly thus would no longer contain much residual suffering to be cleansed in a like manner as was caused by the killer. This is the way with *karma*.

Eat more vegetables and grow up to be a fine child of the divine triplicity, the Mother of Compassion whom we Love.[1] She gave us Life to evolve to progressively higher, enlightened states until Buddhahood is reached. The attainment of Buddhahood necessitates the travelling of the Bodhisattva path. The vow of the Bodhisattva to never cease striving until all sentient beings have been freed from suffering is the way to Buddhahood. This necessitates the protection of animals, of all wild species that grow on the earthy terrain. When you have cleansed enough obstacles on the path of Love, perhaps then you will be freed from the necessity of causing suffering. You will be free and liberated, gone to the other Shore (of being/non-being). Therefore, consume not the consequences of another's suffering, or incarnate again for more education. So be it.

Oṁ! Sarvamaṅgalam - Blessings to All!

---

1   The three sheaths of a Buddha: the Dharmakāya, Sambhogakāya, and Nirmānakāya.

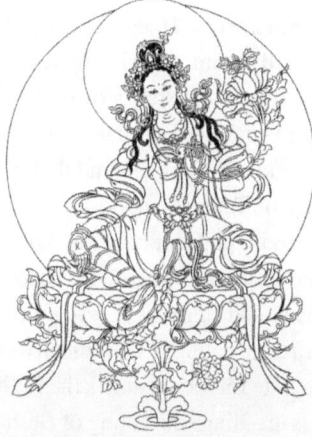

Appendix I

An Extract from *The Laṅkāvatāra Sūtra*

An abstract from chapter eight of Suzuki's translation of: *The Laṅkāvatāra Sūtra*.[1] (Note that this entire chapter concerns itself with the subject of the harmfulness of meat eating.)

At that time Mahāmati the Bodhisattva-Mahāsattva asked the Blessed One in verse and again made a request saying; Pray tell me, Blessed One Tathagata, Arhat, Fully-Enlightened One regarding the merit and vice of meat-eating; thereby I and other Bodhisattva-Mahāsattvas of the present and the future may teach the Dharma to make

---

1   A Mahāyāna text, Translated for the first time from the original Sanskrit by Daisetz Suzuki. (Routledge & Kegan Paul Ltd. 1932, 1973). The extract is taken from pages 211-222.

those beings abandon their greed for meat, who, under the influence
of the habit-energy belonging to the carnivorous existence, strongly
crave meat-food. These meat-eaters thus abandoning their desire for
[its] taste will seek the Dharma for their food and enjoyment, and,
regarding all beings with love as if they were an only child, will cherish
great compassion towards them. Cherishing [great compassion], they
will discipline themselves at the stages of Bodhisattvahood and will
quickly be awakened in supreme enlightenment; or staying a while at
the stage of Śrāvakahood and Pratyekabuddhahood, they will finally
reach the highest stage of Tathagatahood.

Blessed One, even those philosophers who hold erroneous doctrines
and are addicted to the views of the Lokāyata such as dualism of beings
and non-being, nihilism, and eternalism, will prohibit meat-eating, and
will themselves refrain from eating it. How much more, O World Leader,
he who promotes one taste for mercy and is the Fully-Enlightened One;
why not prohibit in his teachings the eating of flesh not only by himself
but by others? Indeed, let the Blessed One who at heart is filled with
pity for the entire world, who regards all beings as his only child, and
who possesses great compassion in compliance with his sympathetic
feelings, teach us as to the merit and vice of meat-eating, so that I and
other Bodhisattva-Mahāsattvas may teach the Dharma.

Said the Blessed One: Then, Mahāmati, listen well and reflect well
within yourself; I will tell you.

Certainly, Blessed One; said Mahāmati the Bodhisattva-Mahāsattva
and gave ear to the Blessed One.

The Blessed One said this to him: For innumerable reasons,
Mahāmati, the Bodhisattvas, whose nature is compassion, is not to
eat any meat; I will explain them Mahāmati, in this long course of
transmigration here, there is not one living being that has not been your
mother, or father, or brother, or sister, or son, or daughter, or the one or
the other, in various degrees of kinship; and when acquiring another
form of life we may live as a beast, as a domestic animal, as a bird,
or as a womb-born, or as something standing in some relationship to
you; [this being so] how can the Bodhisattva-Mahāsattva who desires
to approach all living beings as if they were himself and to practise the
Buddha-truths, eat the flesh of any living being that of the same nature

as himself? Even, Mahāmati, the Kalishasa, listening to the Tathagata's discourse on the highest essence of Dharma, attained the notion of protecting [Buddhism], and, feeling pity, refrains from eating flesh; how much more those who love the Dharma! Thus, Mahāmati, wherever there is the evolution of living beings let people cherish the thought of kinship with them, and thinking that all beings are [to be loved as if they were] an only child, let them refrain from eating meat. So with Bodhisattvas whose nature is compassion, [the eating of] meat is to be avoided by him. Even in exceptional cases it is not [compassionate] of a Bodhisattva of good standing to eat meat. The flesh of a dog, an ass, a buffalo, a horse, a bull, or man, or any other [being], Mahāmati, that is not generally eaten by people, is sold on the roadside as mutton for the sake of money; and therefore, Mahāmati, the Bodhisattva should not eat meat.

For the sake of love of purity, Mahāmati, the Bodhisattva should refrain from eating flesh, which is born of semen, blood, etc. For fear of causing terror to living beings, Mahāmati, let the Bodhisattva, who is disciplining himself to attain compassion, refrain from eating flesh. To illustrate, Mahāmati: When a dog sees, even from a distance, a hunter, a pariah, a fisherman, etc., whose desires are for meat-eating, he is terrified with fear, thinking, "They are death-dealers, they will even kill me." In the same way, Mahāmati, even those minute animals that are living in the air, on earth, and in water, seeing meat-eaters at a distance, will perceive in them, by their keen sense of smell, the odour of the Rakshasa and will run away from such people as quickly as possible, for they are to them the threat of death. For this reason, Mahāmati, let the Bodhisattva, who is disciplining himself, to abide in great compassion, because of its terrifying living beings, refrain from eating meat. Mahāmati, meat which is liked by unwise people is full of bad smell and its eating gives one a bad reputation which turns wise people away; let the Bodhisattva refrain from eating meat. The food of the wise, Mahāmati, is what is eaten by the Rishis; it does not consist of meat and blood. Therefore, Mahāmati, let the Bodhisattva refrain from eating meat.

In order to guard the minds of all people, Mahāmati, let the Bodhisattva whose nature is holy and who is desirous of avoiding censure on the teaching of the Buddha, refrain from eating meat. For instance, Mahāmati, there are some in the world who speak ill of the teaching of the Buddha; [they would say,] "Why are those who are living the life of a Śramaṇa,[2] or a Brahmin reject such food as was enjoyed by the ancient Rishis, and like the carnivorous animals, living in the air, on earth, or in the water? Why do they go wandering about in the world thoroughly terrifying living beings, disregarding the life of a Śramaṇa and destroying the vow of a Brahmin? There is no Dharma, no discipline in them." There are many such adverse-minded people who speak ill of the teaching of the Buddha. For this reason, Mahāmati, in order to guard the minds of all people, let the Bodhisattva whose nature is full of pity and who is desirous of avoiding censure on the teaching of the Buddha, refrain from eating meat.

Mahāmati, there is generally an offensive odour to a corpse, which goes against nature; therefore, let the Bodhisattva refrain from eating meat. Mahāmati, when flesh is burned, whether it be that of a dead man or of some other living creature, there is no distinction of the odour. When flesh of either kind is burned, the odour emitted is equally noxious. Therefore, Mahāmati, let the Bodhisattva, who is ever desirous of purity in his discipline, wholly refrain from eating meat.

Mahāmati, when sons or daughters of good family, wishing to exercise themselves in various disciplines such as the attainment of a compassionate heart, the holding a magical formula, or the perfecting of magical knowledge, or starting on a pilgrimage to the Mahāyāna, retire into a cemetery, or to a wilderness, or a forest, where demons gather or frequently approach; or when they attempt to sit on a couch or seat for the exercise; they are hindered [because of their meat eating] from gaining magical powers or from obtaining emancipation. Mahāmati, seeing that thus there are obstacles to the accomplishing of all the practices, let the Bodhisattva, who is desirous of benefitting himself as well as others, wholly refrain from eating meat.

As even the sight of objective forms gives rise to the desire for tasting their delicious flavour, let the Bodhisattva, whose nature is pity and who regards all beings as his only child, wholly refrain from eating meat. Recognising that his mouth smells most obnoxiously, even

---

2   A monk, mendicant, performing acts of penance and mortification.

while living this life, let the Bodhisattva whose nature is pity, wholly refrain from eating meat.

[The meat-eater[3]] sleeps uneasily and when awakened is distressed. He dreams of dreadful events, which makes his hair rise on end. He is left alone in an empty hut; he leads a solitary life; and his spirit is seized by demons. Frequently he is struck with terror, he trembles without knowing why, there is no regularity in his eating, he is never satisfied. In his eating he never knows what is meant by proper taste, digestion, and nourishment. His viscera are filled with worms and other impure creatures and harbour the cause of leprosy. He ceases to entertain any thoughts of aversion towards all diseases. When I teach to regard food as if it were eating the flesh of one's own child, or taking a drug, how can I permit my disciples, Mahāmati, to eat food consisting of flesh and blood, which is gratifying to the unwise but is abhorred by the wise, which brings many evils and keeps away many merits; and which was not offered to the Rishis and is altogether unsuitable?

Now, Mahāmati, the food I have permitted [my disciples to take] is gratifying to all wise people but is avoided by the unwise; it is productive of many merits, it keeps away many evils; and it has been prescribed by the ancient Rishis. It comprises rice, barley, wheat, kidney beans, lentils, etc.; clarified butter, oil, honey, molasses, treacle, sugar cane, coarse sugar, etc.; food prepared with these is proper food. Mahāmati, there may be some irrational people in the future who will discriminate and establish new rules of moral discipline[4], and who, under the influence of the habit-energy belonging to the carnivorous races, will greedily desire the taste [of meat]: it is not for these people that the above food is prescribed. Mahāmati, this is the food I urge for the Bodhisattva-Mahāsattvas who have made offerings to the previous Buddhas, who have planted roots of goodness, who are all men and women belonging to the Śākya family, who are sons and daughters of good family, who have no attachment to body, life, and property, who do not covet delicacies, are not at all greedy, who being compassionate desire to embrace all

3   Here the Buddha is really referring to the psychic effects of meat eating upon a yogic practitioner of the *dharma*.

4   Such are the modern Buddhists who eat meat toxins and try to justify it somehow upon the basis of quoted scriptures.

living beings as their own person, and who regard all beings with affection as if they were an only child....[5]

If, Mahāmati, meat is not eaten by anybody for any reason, there will be no destroyer of life. Mahāmati, in the majority of cases the slaughtering of innocent living beings is done for pride and very rarely for other causes. Though nothing special may be said of eating the flesh of living creatures such as animals and birds, alas, Mahāmati, that one addicted to the love of [meat-] taste should eat human flesh! Mahāmati, in most cases nets and other devices are prepared in various places by people who have lost their sense on account of their appetite for meat-taste, and thereby many innocent victims are destroyed for the sake of the price [they bring in]—such as birds, Kaurabhraka, Kaivarta, etc., that are moving about in the air, on land, and in water. There are even some, Mahāmati, who are like Rākshasas[6] hard-hearted and used to practising cruelties, who, being so devoid of compassion, would now and then look at living beings as meant for food and destruction—no compassion is awakened in them.

It is not true, Mahāmati, that meat is proper food and permissible when the animal was not killed by himself, when he did not order others to kill it, when it was not specially meant for him. Again, Mahāmati, there may be some unwitted people in the future, who, beginning to lead the homeless life according to my teaching, are acknowledged as sons of the Śākya, and carry the Kāshāya robe about them as a badge, but who are in thought evilly affected by erroneous reasonings. They may talk about various discriminations which they make in their moral discipline, being addicted to the view of a personal soul. Being under the influence of the thirst for [meat-] taste, they will string together in various ways sophistic arguments to defend meat-eating. They think they are giving me an unprecedented calumny when they discriminate and talk about facts that are capable of various interpretations. Imagining that this fact allows this interpretation [they conclude that] the Blessed One permits meat as a proper food, and that it is mentioned among permitted foods and that probably the Tathagata himself partook of it. But, Mahāmati, nowhere in the sutras is meat permitted as some thing

---

5   Here I have omitted a small allegorical section.

6   Demonic beings.

enjoyable, nor is it referred to as proper among the foods prescribed [for the Buddha's followers].

If however, Mahāmati, I had the mind to permit [meat eating], or if I said it was proper for the Śrāvakas[7] [to eat meat], I would not have forbidden, I would not forbid all meat-eating for these Yogins, the sons and daughters of good family, who, wishing to cherish the idea that all beings are to them like an only child, are possessed of compassion, practice contemplation, mortification, and are on their way to the Mahāyāna. And, Mahāmati, the interdiction not to eat any kind of meat is here given to all sons and daughters of good family, whether they are cemetery-ascetics or forest ascetics, or Yogins who are practicing the exercises, if they wish the Dharma and are on the way to the mastery of any vehicle, and being possessed of compassion, conceive the idea of regarding all beings as an only child, in order to accomplish the end of their discipline.

In the canonical texts here and there the practice of discipline is developed in orderly sequence like a ladder going up step by step, and one joined to another in a regular and methodical manner; after explaining each point meat obtained in these specific circumstances is not interdicted. Further, a tenfold prohibition is given as regards the flesh of animals found dead by themselves. But in the present sutra all [meat-eating] in any form, in any manner, and in any place is unconditionally and once for all, prohibited for all. Thus, Mahāmati, meat-eating I have not permitted to anyone, I do not permit, I will not permit. Meat-eating, I tell you, Mahāmati, is not proper for homeless monks. There may be some, Mahāmati, who would say that meat was eaten by the Tathagata thinking this would eliminate him. Such unwitted people as these, Mahāmati, will follow the evil course of their own *karma*-hindrance, and will fall into such regions where long nights are passed without profit and without happiness. Mahāmati, the noble Śrāvakas do not eat the food taken properly by [ordinary] men, how much less the food of flesh and blood, which is altogether improper. Mahāmati, the food for my Śrāvakas, Pratyekabuddhas,[8] and Bodhisattvas is the Dharma

---

7   A 'hearer, listener', a pious attendant to the Buddha, in the Hīnayāna, a disciple, a chela.

8   Each one for himself, individualist Buddha, each one manifesting activity for himself, technically without concern for others. A *pratyekabuddha* is a self-focussed solitary meditator working for Buddhahood.

and not flesh food; how much more the Tathagata! The Tathagata is the Dharmakāya, Mahāmati; he abides in the Dharma as food; his is not a body feeding on flesh; he does not abide in any flesh food. He has ejected the habit-energy of thirst and desire which sustain all existence; he keeps away the habit-energy of all evil passions; he is thoroughly emancipated in mind and knowledge; he is the All-knower; he is All-seer; he regards all beings impartially as an only child; he is a great compassionate heart. Mahāmati, having the thought of an only child for all beings, how can I, such as I am, permit the Śrāvakas to eat the flesh of their own child? How much less my eating it! That I have permitted the Śrāvakas as well as myself to partake of [meat-eating], Mahāmati, has no foundation whatever.

So it is said:

1. Liquor, meat, and onions are to be avoided, Mahāmati, by the Bodhisattva-Mahāsattvas and those who are Victor-heroes.

2. Meat is not agreeable to the wise: it has a nauseating odour, it causes a bad reputation, it is food for the carnivorous; I say this, Mahāmati, it is not to be eaten.

3. To those who eat [meat] there are detrimental effects, to those who do not, merits; Mahāmati, you should know that meat-eaters bring detrimental effects upon themselves.

4. Let the Yogin refrain from eating flesh as it is born of himself, as [the eating] involves transgression, as [flesh] is produced of semen and blood, and as [the killing of animals] causes terror to living beings.

5. Let the Yogin always refrain from meat, onion, various kinds of liquor, allium and garlic.[9]

6. Do not anoint the body with sesamum oil; do not sleep on a bed perforated with spikes; for the living beings who find shelter in the cavities and in places where there are no cavities may be terribly frightened.[10]

---

9   Onion and garlic is included in this list because they produce a disagreeable odour, but can be included in the listing of permissible substances for yogins, because the effects are easily transmuted, however liqour and mind altering drugs, not so because of the effect they have upon consciousness and the psychic constitution.

10   Suzuki states in a footnote that this is 'Unintelligible as far as the translator can see'.

7. From eating [meat] arrogance is born, from arrogance erroneous imaginations issue, and from imagination is born greed; and for this reason refrain from eating [meat].

8. From imagination greed is born, and by greed the mind is stupefied; there is attachment to stupefaction and there is no emancipation from birth [and death].

9. For profit sentient beings are destroyed, for flesh money is paid out, they are both evil-doers and [the dead] matures in the hells called Raurava (screaming), etc.

10. One who eats flesh, trespassing against the word of the Muni, is evil-minded; he is pointed out in the writings of the Śākya as the destroyer of the welfare of the two worlds.

11. These evil-doers go to the most horrifying hell, meat-eaters are matured in the terrific hells such as Raurava, etc.

12. There is no meat to be regarded as pure in three ways: not premeditated, not asked for, and not impelled, therefore, refrain from eating meat.

13. Let not the Yogin eat meat, it is forbidden by myself as well as by the Buddhas; those sentient beings who feed on one another will be reborn among the carnivorous animals.

14. [The meat-eater] is ill-smelling, contemptuous, and born deprived of intelligence; he will be born again among the families of the Caṇḍāla, the Pukkasa, and the Domba.

15. From the womb of Ḍākinī he will be born in the meat eaters' family, and then into the womb of a Rākshasī and a cat; he belongs to the lowest class of men.

16. Meat-eating is rejected by me in such sutras as the *Hastikakshya*, the *Mahāmegha*, the *Nirvāna*, the *Aṅglimālika*, and the *Laṅkāvatāra*.

17. [Meat-eating] is condemned by the Buddhas, Bodhisattvas, and Śrāvakas; if one devours [meat] out of shamelessness he will always be devoid of sense.

18. One who avoids meat, etc., will be born, because of this fact, in the family of the Brahmins or of the Yogins, endowed with knowledge and wealth.

19. Let one avoid all meat-eating [whatever they may say about] witnessing, hearing, and suspecting; these theorisers born in a carnivorous family understand this not.

20. As greed is the hindrance to emancipation, so are meat eating, liquor, etc., hindrances.

21. There may be in time to come people who make foolish remarks about meat-eating; saying, 'Meat is proper to eat, unobjectionable, and permitted by the Buddha."

22. Meat-eating is a medicine; again, it is like a child's flesh; follow the proper measure and be averse [to meat, and thus] let the Yogin go about begging.

23. [Meat-eating] is forbidden by me everywhere and all the time for those who are abiding in compassion; [he who eats meat] will be born in the same place as the lion, tiger, wolf, etc.

24. Therefore, do not eat meat which will cause terror among people, because it hinders the truth of emancipation; [not to eat meat—] this is the mark of the wise.

Here Ends the Eighth Chapter, "On Meat-eating," from the *Laṅkāvatāra*, the "Essence of the Teaching of All the Buddhas".

Appendix II

A Brief Exposition on the Nature of *Karma*

Translated literally, the Sanskrit term *karma* means action, which then produces reaction. It is the great law of cause and effect, for no matter what actions one sows in the three worlds of human livingness (or non-actions, when one should have acted), one must reap the consequence of their effects.

One reaps the consequence of not only one's physical actions, but also of one's emotional and mental life, and of non-action and non-involvement when one had the ability to help. One's *karma* is one's destiny, and beings with interrelated *karma* from another earlier epoch of existence incarnate together in order to work out their *karma*. This means that there are certain actions from the past that must be rectified or cleansed by the perpetuators. If someone caused harm or pain to another in the past by not acting when clearly they should have, then there was *karma* created. An example is if a person who cannot swim has fallen into deep water and is in danger of drowning with someone who can swim in the vicinity, then the situation has been karmically designed for him/her to jump in and save that person. If the person does not act to save the drowning person, which so easily could have been done, then the *karma* of the sum of the prospective future actions of the person drowning weighs upon the one who did not act to save.

Another way of looking at this is thus: What would be the consequences of a great one, such as Milarepa, or the Buddha, who clearly had the *karma* and spiritual gift waves from past actions to gain enlightenment (indeed, whose *karma* necessitated it), who at a crucial moment decided that the going was too tough? Perhaps they decided to be a fisherman instead? Certainly in such a case the sum of those they did not help would be great. (Indeed those who had the good *karma* with these great beings to have incarnated precisely to be taught by them would also not gain their enlightenment.) Perhaps falling thus also into a cycle of doing unmeritorious deeds. The sum of the *karma* of all of the subsequent wrong actions (rippling out through to the many they could have helped) becomes the *karma* of the one who was destined to be Buddha, Milarepa, in that life. As for great ones, so it is similarly for those not so highly attained. There are always certain actions that one is predestined to do, and one is impelled to do so according to the way one's conscience (or as the 'Voice of Silence') dictates. People have to learn to rightly listen to that voice throughout their lives.

Karma, however, is not absolutely fixed. For example, one can consciously choose to not act in accordance with the way one should. Thus they will create new *karma,* a new score to cleanse through reciprocal action in a future time.

Karma is concerned with the means by which consciousness evolves. It is gauged on the objective and subjective *motives* underlying the actions of the being, as well as the consequences of the actions. It is the law of perpetual fulfilment. The being, through the consequences of his/her actions and the resultant suffering or happiness, is eventually impelled to transmute their grosser tastes into the refined and subtle.

Desires turn into aspirations; petty and selfish ambitions blossom into the selfless expression of the *dharma;* ignorance evolves into wisdom; darkness is transmuted into (a resplendent vehicle of) Love and Light.

Karma is primarily a group law and thus affects all civilisations, nations, races, and kingdoms of Nature. Nobody lives separate from anyone else – all thoughts, emotions and physical actions happen in context with their relationship to others. Indeed, the way one thinks and the language one uses are a consequence of being part of a society in a particular country in a particular era of human history. Everyone in that society conditions the way the others think and feel. Consequently, the *karma* is interwoven, thus explaining why it is a group law. People come into and out of incarnation according to the *karma* of their subjective group. This *karma* prompts masses of people toward certain events. People live in a sea of conditionings that constitute their *karma,* and it is this that urges them towards fulfilment.

Karma, therefore, is the cause and effect of the purpose for the existence of any evolving entity. Its real nature is thus inexplicable to the thinking minds of people. They can be considered as atoms constituting a grain of sand, karmically propelled in the immense duration of cosmos.

In conjunction with cyclic law, *karma* is the prime underlying cause of all natural disasters, wars, and yet also causes the beneficial effects of, for example, rain and sunshine. This is because all aspects of manifest life are expressions of *karma.*

The objective of *karma* in its seemingly destructive aspect is the disintegration of an old form, so as to birth a new form that can adequately and effectively wield a higher type of energy. This signifies a truer or more comprehensive aspect that would have been distorted by the old, rigid, or limited expression.

A liberated being is one who has no more *karma* left associated with the material world, the *three realms* of perception where humanity has its being. (The qualities of which we must learn to perfectly control and express.) These are the dense physical, emotional, and the mental realms (with its dual aspects of the concrete and abstract Mind).

When liberated beings continue to be involved with the material world, it is entirely for compassionate reasons and to help anchor the new type of *karma* (which may be termed planetary *karma)* that now manifests through them.

All of a person's pain (or joy) can thus be viewed as self-caused. Basically, the formula is - if a person thinks only of themselves and thus is separative (taking from all others to satisfy the desires of the self), then inevitably *karma* rebounds upon that person to take from them that which is cherished as 'self'. (With the consequent pain that frustrated personality ambition produces.)

If a person thinks of others as themselves, and gives to them with his/her heart, then the link with the Source of all Light and Love is increased, with consequent joy. Thus as the Heart grows with Love and Light, so too does the *karma* expand to affect groups, nations, and eventually the entire world with the Power of Light, as many great enlightened beings have shown.

Karma can also be viewed in terms of the point of view of two of the basic postulates of physics, which are:

a. Energy can be neither created nor destroyed – it is only transmuted from one state to the next.

b. Newton's third law states – mutual reactions between two bodies produce equal and opposite reactions; or, to every action there is always an equal and opposite reaction.

The 'equal and opposite reaction', therefore, is the *karma* that we incur for ourselves by our actions. It is opposite in that the consequences are relayed back to us in a similar fashion to a mirror image. There is nothing created or destroyed, only the forms are changed or modified to suit the needs of the various evolving external conditionings, or environment.

The consequences of the actions of people unfailingly manifest in such a way that they grow in experience, allowing them to mature spiritually. For this reason, they are made to realise the extent of those consequences by living them fully in consciousness.

No one can evade these consequences, nor can any compassionate being relieve another person from experiencing the weight of their *karma* until such a time as that person realises the cause of these sufferings for themselves, and takes the first step towards Light. Then, and only then, can they be helped, for only what people have experienced for themselves can be known and become an integral part of their being.

Appendix III

The Factor of Meat Eating

In the accounts below I shall share some of the vast amount of information and examples that could be presented concerning the inhumanity of the present day meat industry. Very few people actually understand the circumstances of meat production and the wider impact it has on the environment and the underprivileged world.

Meat production is at the heart of almost every environmental disaster confronting the earth, from deforestation to desertification, global warming and acid rain. Soil erosion, loss of habitat and water depletion – the causes of which are all deeply ingrained in the need for meat. Below is presented a small select portion of the information of the type that all concerned people should be aware of. Much more could have been presented, but the educated reader can research further pertinent (and maybe more up to date) facts for themselves.

- One third of the 150 acres of rainforest destroyed each day is for cattle grazing.[1]

- Just one quarter-pound hamburger requires the clearing of fifty-five square yards of rain forest and the destruction of one hundred and sixty five pounds of living matter, including twenty to thirty different plant species, one hundred insect species, and dozens of bird, mammal, and reptile species.[2]

- Commercial fishing has caused almost two-thirds of the world's oceans to clamour on the edges of survival.[3]

- Livestock production uses immense portions of the world's resources in highly inefficient and wasteful ways.

- Four-fifths of the world's agricultural land is used for feeding animals and one-fifth for feeding man directly.[4]

- Animals need 20 pounds of protein for every pound they yield as meat.

- An acre of walnuts will supply twenty times the amount of protein the same acre would yield in beef.[5]

- Twenty pure vegetarians can be fed on the amount of land needed to feed one person consuming a meat-based diet.[6]

- Mixed vegetable proteins are of a better quality than meat products because they contain vegetable *prāṇas* and vitality. It is only due to ignorance (along with the powerful influence of the meat industry, working in unison with man's desire for flesh) that people have chosen to ignore the superior values in nuts and pulses.

1 *Sierra*, March 1995, p. 26.

2 Julie Denslow and Christine Padoch, *People of the Tropical Rainforest* (Berkeley: University of California Press. 1988), 169.

3 Juliet Gellatley with Tony Wardle, *The Silent Ark,* (Thorsons, 2000).

4 Wynne-Tyson,Jon, *Food for a Future, The Ecological Priority of a Humane Diet*, (Abacus, 1976), 16.

5 Ibid.

6 British Meat, *49 Reasons to go Vegetarian,* www.britishmeat.com/49.htm, November 10, 1999.

• The inefficient use of land resources involved with the production of meat for food causes the poverty and hunger that we see throughout the world today. If adopted world wide, plant protein could play a huge part in solving the world's hunger problems.

• Chronic hunger and related disease affect more than 1.3 billion people. Never before in human history has such a large percentage of our species—more than 20 percent—been undernourished, [7] yet one third of the world's total grain harvest is fed to cattle and other livestock.[8]

• The world's cattle alone, not to mention pigs and chickens, consume a quantity of food equal to the caloric needs of 8.7 billion people.[9]

• Third world countries grain yields are shipped to feed the cattle in America. If worldwide agricultural production were shifted from livestock feed to food grains for direct human consumption, more than a billion people could be fed – the precise number which currently suffer from hunger and malnourishment.[10]

• To a compassionate mind that truly contemplates the suffering of others, one cannot partake in an industry that causes such an inhumane distribution of resources upon this planet. Millions of people starve whilst chickens are overfed to such an extent that their legs break under the strain of massively disproportionate weight.

• Fertile lands are turned into arid and barren deserts due to cattle farming. The intensive grazing involved in this process causes soil erosion and nutrient depletion, which harms plant life (and in some cases, renders the soil totally infertile). Lifeless deserts are gradually filling our earth, where previously the land was rich with life. This is called desertification.

---

7   Myra Klockenbrinli, *The New Range War Has the Desert As Foe*, (New York Times. August 20, 1991).

8   Catherine Caulfield, *A Reporter at Large: The Rain Forests*, (New Yorker, January 14, 1985), 79.

9   Rensberger, p. 14.

10   *The Vegetarian Times*, November 1994, p. 100.

- The meat industry is also a very generous contributor to the 'greenhouse effect', the major cause of the current slight warming of the planet, denoted by some alarmists to be the harbinger of a major climate crisis known as global warming.[11] Cattle and beef production is a significant factor in the emission of three of the four 'global warming' gases—carbon dioxide, nitrous oxide, and methane.[12]

- Much of the carbon dioxide released into the atmosphere is directly attributable to beef production: burning forests to make way for cattle pasture and burning massive tracts of agricultural waste from cattle feed crops. When the fifty-five square feet of rain forest needed to produce one quarter-pound hamburger is burned for pasture, 500 pounds of carbon dioxide is released into the atmosphere.[13]

- More than 90 billion animals die yearly for human consumption.[14] As previously mentioned, the methods of slaughter are oft barbaric and cruel.

- Many food animals are killed by the process of Kosher slaughter. Kosher slaughter involves hanging an animal, particularly a cow or pig, by its hooves. The animal's neck is cut without any kind of anaesthesia. The animal hangs and bleeds to death.

---

11   The issue of global warming (now known as 'climate change') is quite contentious and overhyped. The climate changes all of the time, whilst the sun is the major contributing factor behind real climate change momentums, rather than anything caused by human action (such as the increase of CO_2 levels). There is faulty 'science' behind the 'climate change' hype. We are in fact in an inter-glacial period, and the climate could just as well be headed towards another major glacial period. One just needs to witness the huge climate swings (that vastly dwarf anything seen nowadays) during the Younger Dryas period (11 – 13,000 years ago) and earlier, to see the fallacy of the presented hype. There were no modern humans with their technological activities then.

12   Fred Pearce, *Methane: The Hidden Greenhouse Gas,* (New Scientist, May 6, 1989).

13   *Greenhouse Crisis Statistical Review,* Sources: World Resources Institute, Rainforest Action Network. U.S. Department of Agriculture. and World Watch Institute in U.S. News and World Report, Oct 31, 1988.

14   The Vegan Option: *A Look at Non-violent Eating,* www.cok-online.org/literature/vegan_option.html, 1999. In relation to the 90 billion animals slaughtered, see also: https://ourworldindata.org/how-many-animals-get-slaughtered-every-day

- Another method of slaughter is by a man wielding a poleax (a type of axe), standing above the animal, and then trying to knock it unconscious with a single blow. The problem is that he must aim a long overhead swing at a moving target; to succeed, the hammer must land at a precise point on the animal's head, and a frightened animal is quite likely to move its head. If the swing is a fraction astray, the hammer can crash through the animal's eye or nose; then, as the animal thrashes around in agony and terror, several more blows may be needed to knock it unconscious.[15]

Chickens

Many birds are killed while fully conscious; others are shocked with electricity at 12.5 mA, which paralyses them and allows for easier feather release. However, it would take 120 mA to render them unconscious. The birds are hung upside down from a conveyor belt and their throats are cut (by a human or a machine). Occasionally, a bird will break free and be left to die thrashing in pools of blood on the floor. Birds who do not bleed to death before they reach the scalding tank are boiled alive.[16]

This gory process brings an end to a very unhappy life. The conditions of life for an animal in the West today, especially with the boom of 'factory farming', are filled with unimaginable pain.

Factory hens today are forced to live in "battery" cages stacked in rows, four high, by the thousands. Each will be confined to about 48 square inches of space. After months of confinement, necks will be covered with blisters, wings bare, combs bloody, feet torn. Manure fumes and rotting carcasses will force poultry workers to wear gas masks. When the hens have become what the industry matter-of-factly refers to as 'spent', producers will truck the mutilated birds—often long distances--to slaughter (or they will gas them, or grind them up while still alive, to be used as feed for the next flock).[17]

---

15 Peter Singer, *Animal Liberation,* New York: (New York Review: Avon, 1975), 160-1.

16 The Vegan Society.

17 Pamela Rice, *101 Reasons to be Vegetarian,* (The Viva Vegie Society New York 1999, No 16).

Factory farmers sear off the beaks of all laying hens shortly after birth, a painful procedure performed without anaesthesia. Each year, laying hens hatch more than 400 million chicks, half of whom are males. Only female chicks are of use to the egg industry, so every male chick born to a laying hen is killed on his day of birth. The two most common methods of slaughter for male chicks are grinding them alive or simply throwing them into garbage bags while still living, only to suffocate under the weight of other male chicks.

'Broilers', the other type of factory-farmed chicken, are raised for their flesh, not eggs. 90 percent of broilers have trouble walking because of their huge weight. These birds have been bred to grow twice as large at twice the rate as 'traditional' chickens. All are slaughtered after only seven weeks of life.[18]

Cows

Some modern dairy cows are rarely, if ever, allowed out of their stall, are milked up to three times a day and are kept pregnant nearly all of their abbreviated life. Their calves are taken from them within hours of birth to prevent the calf from drinking milk.[19] A cow often cries out and searches for its calf for days after it is taken away.[20]

The almost constant pregnancies and obscene milk yields create dairy cows who are chronically ill. Each year, tens of thousands of dairy cows become too weak or ill to even stand. Naturally, cows live about 20 years. Modern dairy cows become so worn down that they are slaughtered at age five. As if the pain of having her child ripped from her at birth is not enough, the typical modern dairy cow will spend most of her life standing in a concrete stall.

If the calf is male, he will be ripped from his mother and sold to a veal farm during his first day or so of life.[21]

18   The Vegan Option: *A Look at Non-violent Eating,* www.cok-online.org/literature/vegan_option.html, 1999.

19   *The Vegan Outreach*

20   Wynne-Tyson, Jon, *Food for a Future - The Ecological Priority of a Humane Diet,* (Abacus, 1976), 109-11.

21   USDA, Animal and Plant Health Inspection Service, Dairy Heifer Morbidity, Mortality, and Health Management Focusing on Preweaned (Fort Collins, CO, Feb.

On veal farms, calves spend their entire lives chained inside a crate too small for them to even turn around in. To keep their flesh pale and soft, they are fed an iron-deficient diet (causing anaemia) and are kept virtually motionless for the entirety of their short lives. They will never feel the grass in a paddock, or suckle from their mothers. After 16 weeks of intense confinement, barely able to walk, veal calves are unchained and sent to slaughter.

Veal calves are so sick that antibiotics and other drugs are routinely used to keep as many of them alive as possible until their slaughter.[22]

A calf is prodded and dragged into the killing pen, wide-eyed and terrified with the stench of blood and death in its nostrils. When the captive bolt shatters its forehead there is no compassion. When the slaughterer's hand grabs the muzzle of a lamb to stifle its bleating and applies the knife to its throat, there is no compassion.[23]

Pigs and Sheep

To reduce labour costs, pigs live on concrete slats as flooring. The animals literally never touch earth during the four months they spend growing to 'slaughter weight'. The only movement furrowing crates allow is about one step backward and one step forward. The boredom and constant confinement drive sows to insanity, causing stereotypic behaviour such as pacing back and forth and biting the bars that imprison them.

'Forget the pig is an animal. Treat him just like a machine in a factory.' - Hog Farm Management

Spinal columns of conscious sheep are severed with the probing of a domestic screwdriver; paralysed bullocks urged to stand with 70,000 volt shocks to the testicles; fully conscious lambs slashed across the throat because time is of the essence.[24]

1994), 16.

22 Mason and Singer, *Animal Factories*, 81-89.

23 Juliet Gellatley with Tony Wardle, *The Silent Ark*, (Thorsons, 2000).

24 Ibid.

British Meat Ingredients List

Just for a tasty aperitif, here are the true ingredients in your next meat dish:

Rat faeces; cow urine; cow pus; tranquilisers; ground up cow heads ('puke heads' contaminated with hair, dirt, and ingest); chicken and cow manure (a 'beef fattener' with e-coli contamination); 'rendered' cows and sheep (recycled animal parts, diseased 'downers' and road kills added to anima feed); euthanised animals from human societies, etc.; growth steroid hormones (fatteners); radioactive isotopes; antibiotics (disease controllers); pesticides; herbicides; insecticides; larvicides; lethal euthanasia drugs such as sodium phenobarbital; a host of diseases from the cow, including pneumonia, bovine aids and perhaps mad cow chemicals like phosphorous to mask putrefaction; various carcinogenic chemicals, including dioxin (one of most deadly known chemicals, also present in Agent Orange).[25]

Food from animals contain their waste, including adrenalin, uric and lactic acid, etc. Before adding ketchup, the biggest contributors to the 'flavour profile' of a hamburger are the leftover blood and urine.[26]

If these compassionate considerations are meaningful to you, then reconsider your meat eating and become vegetarian. The *karma* of animal slaughter is immense. The killing must stop.

---

25 *British Meat*, britishmeat.com, 2000.

26 *The Whole Earth Vegetarian Catalogue.*

Appendix IV

Levels of Tantra[1]

Vajrayāna practices, or Tantric teachings, have been systematised into four categories, and practitioners are encouraged to follow the Tantric teachings in a systematic and gradual way. The relationship that exists between the visualised deities and the practitioner will go through different transitions, depending upon the level of Tantra with which the person engages. Even the natures of the visualised deities are different; they may be wrathful or peaceful, for example. The four basic levels generally represented are:

---

1   This section has been adapted mainly from information presented courtesy of LM at the Kargyu email group.

Kriya Tantra

The first level of Tantra is Kriya Tantra, or Action Tantra. The practice of Kriya Tantra emphasises rituals, which are very important....Three different Buddha families are mentioned on the level of Kriya Tantra: the Padma, or Lotus family; the Vajra family, and the family of the Buddhas....At the Kriya Tantra level, the relationship between the practitioner and the deity is essentially one of inequality. We see ourselves as being deluded, while the deity is worshipped as having all the power to impart to us.

Charya Tantra

The practitioner then proceeds to the next stage, which is Charya Tantra, or Performance Tantra. Charya Tantra emphasises the importance of both meditative states and ritual observances....When one practices the visualisation of deities on the level of Charya Tantra, it is no longer based upon the same sense of inequality that defined Kriya Tantra. The deities are seen more as friends than exalted beings to be worshiped, even while having nothing in common with the practitioner in terms of qualities....In Charya Tantra, the deities are visualised as having two aspects, relative and absolute....The absolute nature of the visualised deities is understood to be no different from one's own Buddha-nature, or the nature of mind. The basic point is that the visualisation of the deities is not absolute, because the deities are a projection of the mind.

Anuyoga Tantra

From Charya Tantra one moves onto the next level, which is Anuyoga Tantra, or Union Tantra, being chiefly concerned with internal visualisation. On this level, one relies less and less on relative truth and aims more toward absolute truth....On the Anuyoga Tantric level, it is said that one must have developed *bodhichitta* and taken the Bodhisattva vow, for without it one cannot continue the practice. Anuyoga Tantra practice involves dealing with delusions and defilements directly, so that they can become transformed into the five wisdoms....When understood properly, these very delusions can be transformed into wisdom, and therefore the delusions are the very material that constitutes what we mean by wisdom....One does not make a sharp distinction between what should be abandoned and what should be cultivated. If one knows how to deal with things that normally give rise to delusions, one can, in fact, give rise to insight and wisdom instead...

Supreme Yoga Tantra

The final level of Tantra, Anuttarayoga Tantra is considered to be the supreme level. It is also the most difficult one to practice. These Tantras look to the original nature of the mind in its primordial purity, its naturalness in space. All deities are seen in complete fusion with their consorts (whether peaceful or wrathful), signifying the ultimate attainment of the highest wisdom born out of *śūnyatā*.

Oṁ

Bibliography

Balsys, Bodo. *A Treatise on Mind, Volume 1.* Sydney: Universal
Dharma Publishing, 2016.

——. *A Treatise on Mind, Volume 5A.* Sydney: Universal Dharma
Publishing, 2015.

——. *A Treatise on Mind, Volume 5B.* Sydney: Universal Dharma
Publishing, 2015.

——. *A Treatise on Mind, Volume 6.* Sydney: Universal Dharma
Publishing, 2014.

——. *A Treatise on Mind, Volume 7A.* Sydney: Universal Dharma
Publishing, 2017.

——. *A Treatise on Mind, Volume 7B&C.* Sydney: Universal Dharma
Publishing, 2018.

——. *Karma and the Rebirth of Consciousness.* Delhi: Munshiram
Manoharlal, 2006.

——. *The Revelation, Revised Edition.* Sydney: Universal Dharma
Publishing, 2022.

Cayley, Vyvyan (Ed.). *The Life of the Mahāsiddha Tilopa.* Dharamsala:
Library of Tibetan Works and Archives, 1995.

Chomsky, Noam and Marv Waterstone. *Consequences of Capitalism:
Manufacturing discontent and resistance.* Chicago: Haymarket
Books, 2021.

Cowell, E. B. (Ed.), *The Jataka Tales.* In five volumes, sacred-texts.
com, January, 2006.

Daisetz Suzuki, *The Laṅkāvatāra Sūtra.* London: Routledge & Kegan Paul Ltd. 1973.

Denslow, Julie and Christine Padoch. *People of the Tropical Rainforest.* Berkeley: University of California Press. 1988.

Evans-Wentz, W.Y. *Tibetan Yoga and Secret Doctrines.* London: Oxford University Press, 1982.

——. *Tibet's Great Yogī Milarepa.* London: Oxford University Press, 1969.

Gellatley, Juliet with Tony Wardle. *The Silent Ark.* Thorsons, 1996.

Geshe Kelsang Gyatso. *Clear Light of Bliss. Mahamudra in Vajrayana Buddhism.* Boston: Wisdom Publications, 1982.

Goddard, Dwight, Ed. *A Buddhist Bible.* Dutton. New York: 1952.

Guenther, Herbert V. *The Life and Teachings of Naropa.* Boston: Shambhala Publications, Inc., 1986.

Govinda, Lama Anagarika. *Foundations of Tibetan Mysticism.* New York: Samuel Weiser, 1975.

Kapleau, Roshi Philip, *To Cherish all Life.* The Zen Centre, Inc., 1981.

King James Version of the Bible (KJV). London: Oxford University Press.

Prashad, Brahmcahri Sital. India: *A Comparative Study of Jainism and Buddhism.* Delhi: Sri Satguru Publications, 1982.

Wynne-Tyson, Jon. *Food for a Future.* The Ecological Priority of a Humane Diet. Abacus, 1976.

Journals and magazines and internet links:

British Meat, britishmeat.com, 2000.

British Meat, *49 Reasons to go Vegetarian,* www.britishmeat.com/49. htm, November 10, 1999.

Caulfield, Catherine. *A Reporter at Large: The Rain Forests,* (New Yorker, January 14, 1985.

Greenhouse Crisis Statistical Review, Sources: World Resources Institute, Rainforest Action Network. U.S. Department of Agriculture. and World Watch Institute in U.S. News and World Report, Oct 31, 1988.

Klockenbrinli, Myra. *The New Range War Has the Desert As Foe.* New York Times. August 20, 1991.

LM at the Kargyu email group.

Mason and Singer, *Animal Factories*.

Mothering, Fall 1996,

Pearce, Fred. *Methane: The Hidden Greenhouse Gas*. New Scientist, May 6, 1989.

Rice, Pamela, *101 Reasons to be Vegetarian*. The Viva Vegie Society New York 1999, No 16.

Sierra, March 1995.

Singer, Peter, *Animal Liberation,* New York Review: Avon, 1975.

The Vegan Option: *A Look at Non-violent Eating,* www.cok-online.org/ literature/vegan_option.html, 1999. In relation to the 90 billion animals slaughtered

[See also: https://ourworldindata.org/how-many-animals-get- slaughtered-every-day]

The Vegan Society.

The Vegan Outreach

The Vegetarian Times, November 1994.

USDA, Animal and Plant Health Inspection Service, Dairy Heifer Morbidity, Mortality, and Health Management Focusing on Preweaned (Fort Collins, CO, Feb. 1994), 16.

The Whole Earth Vegetarian Catalogue.

Index

About the Author

BODO BALSYS is the founder of The School of Esoteric Sciences. He is an author of many books on subjects centred on Buddhism and the Esoteric Sciences, a meditation teacher, poet, artist, spiritual scientist and healer. He has studied extensively across multiple traditions including Esoteric Science, Buddhism, Christianity, Esoteric Healing, Western Science, Art, Politics and History. His advanced esoteric insights, gained through decades of meditative contemplation, enable him to provide a rich understanding of the spiritual pathway toward enlightenment, healing and service.

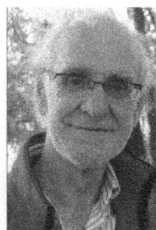

Bodo's teachings can be accessed via the School of Esoteric Science's website:
http://universaldharma.com

For any other enquiries, please email
sangha@universaldharma.com

About Universal Dharma Publishing

Universal Dharma Publishing is a not for profit publisher. Our aim is make innovative, original and esoteric spiritual teachings accessible to all who genuinely aspire to awaken and serve humanity. The books published aim in part to provide an esoteric interpretation of the meaning of Buddhist *dharma* with view of reformation of the way people perceive the meaning of the related teachings. Hopefully then Buddhism can more effectively serve its principal function as a vehicle for enlightenment, and further prosper into the future. A further aim is to provide the next level of exposition of the esoteric doctrines to be revealed to humanity following on the wisdom tradition pioneered by H.P. Blavatsky and A.A. Bailey.

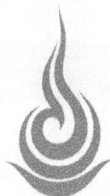

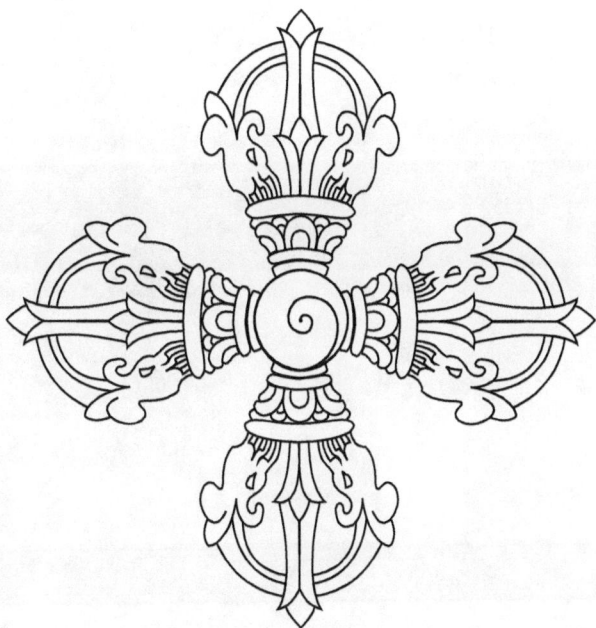

www.ingramcontent.com/pod-product-compliance
Lightning Source LLC
Chambersburg PA
CBHW020355270326
41926CB00007B/446